A BRAIN'S BATTLE AGAINST A STROKE

My recovery combines my memories of Dad's approach with Medicine Today

ROBERT SUSSLER

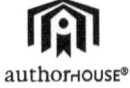

authorHOUSE®

AuthorHouse™
1663 Liberty Drive
Bloomington, IN 47403
www.authorhouse.com
Phone: 1-800-839-8640

First published by AuthorHouse 12/13/2010

ISBN: 978-1-4259-9785-4 (sc)
ISBN: 978-1-4259-9784-7 (dj)
ISBN: 978-1-4343-1536-6 (e)

Library of Congress Control Number: 2007901869

Printed in the United States of America

This book is printed on acid-free paper.

Certain stock imagery © Thinkstock.

This book is dedicated to Dr. David Sussler, my father who practiced medicine from 1919 to 1973, and to Dr. Louis Caplan, Professor of Neurology at Harvard Medical School-- two physicians who combined the best skills using the available science of medicine with a keen insight into how to motivate the patient.

Table of Contents

Preface

This book is the story of my battle to recover from a stroke. My partial recovery combined the skills of modern medicine with my memories about how my dad practiced medicine fifty years earlier. These earlier memories recalled that my dad treated the whole patient. Not until one year after the stroke did a neurologist take the time to get inside of me as a human being as well as focus on my physical injuries. From that time forward I had the daily determination to fight my own brain and to maximize my recovery.

The book will help stroke suffers to overcome the brain damage caused by the stroke. The book will make physician specialists more aware of the need to treat the patient as a person as well as the beneficiary of their specialty skills.

My long term memory allows the readers to find themselves practicing medicine fifty years ago. They will experience my hospitalization after my stroke, and the difficulties I had adjusting to a partial recovery.

The specialists used the available technologies at a large hospital to try to discover the cause of my stroke but they were not able to establish the reason for the blood clots that stopped the flow of blood to minute tissues within two sections of the brain. The neurologists prescribed a pharmaceutical, coumadin, to thin my blood to reduce the danger of another stroke and a medicine, tramadol, to reduce pain to alleviate my discomfort.

Each specialist was competent within the knowledge of his specialty. Each specialty, the neurologists, the internist, the cardiologist, and the hematologist used the latest technology, the science of medicine, as part of their skills. In their brief visits with me I would hear an update of their medical findings.

In the period 50 years earlier when my dad practiced medicine, there was the necessity to diagnosis through a verbal exchange with the patient and to motivate the patient and the family. Physicians lacked both technology and pharmaceuticals.

The descriptive material about each era of medical practice and the relationship between the physician and the patient is based on my personal experiences together with interviews and research.

To augment my primary sources of knowledge, I researched the curriculum of medical schools during each period and read books and articles about the history of United States medicine. Interviews provided additional exposure both with patients of my dad whose memories could recall experiences fifty years previous, with physicians who knew my dad, and with physician specialists involved in the current practice of medicine.

My personal experiences set out a vivid picture. Fifty years ago with less scientific tools, medicine treated the whole patient. The patient was an important part of the curing process. The reader learns that there is a tendency now to treat only the medical problem with advanced scientific tools and the multitude of drugs. In both eras of practice physicians used the available scientific knowledge to try to provide the best care for a patient.

Today enough time may not be available with the patient to focus on the patient's attitude and understanding as well as that of the family's. Both the patient and the family are important to maximize a recovery. The physician specialists practicing medicine today often use technology and pharmaceuticals as better curing tools than the motivation of the patient and the family.

This book illustrates the need to treat the whole patient because of the importance of a patient 's knowledge and attitude in many recoveries. This book can help physicians to understand the need to treat not only the injury or illness but the patient as a person The book provides important insights of the need for a patient and the family to join together in the curing and recovery. They need to understand both the pathological and psychological damages caused by a stroke that results in permanent disability.

As a financial attorney who suffered permanent disability while still active in my profession, I was able to use my professional training to organize the details of my exposure to modern medicine. I combined this exposure with my memories from childhood to write a moving and informative book.

My Stroke

I was sitting comfortably on a soft cushioned chair in the upstairs study. The front windows facing east gave me a view of Long Island Sound. At eight I turned on the television set to watch my Friday night entertainment. The clouds in the sky reflected a reddish glow from the sun beyond the western horizon.

I had enjoyed a mussel and linguini dinner. My wife, Ruth, was busy in the kitchen putting plates and glasses in the dishwasher.I had changed from a gray conservatively tailored suit to light tan slacks. My tie was back in the rack. I had taken off my shoes and put on my Chinese made brown cotton slippers. Memorial day was two weeks away when I would begin to give serious thought to swimming in the Sound The water temperature had to read 62 degrees or higher. On weekends I played tennis.

On April 19, 1992 I had celebrated my 64th birthday. My regular yearly physical revealed no underlying health concerns. I was trying to reduce my professional work load so that my legal career could continue beyond normal retirement, a plan for the future.

My dad had practiced medicine until he was 83. At age 100 he could walk unassisted. His mind was alert and full of memories. Until the end of his practice he had been my only doctor. I had had the usual childhood illnesses. My most serious illness was a severe case of influenza at age forty six. My only treatment at a hospital was when I was born.

My professional life till 1982 had included many years in which

I had commuted from New London to Hartford driving the hour that it took to reach my office from the sea shore.My early career involved complicated commercial real estate transactions. Because of the cyclical period of high interest rates making mortgage financing difficult, I had studied utility rate making to represent consumers. I lobbied and created the first Cooperative utility in Connecticut.I filed anti trust suits against Northeast Utilities to open up the right for the Cooperative to own its own generation and for cities to buy their street lightening rather than pay only a leasing rate. The earnings from the utility practice supplemented any contraction in my Real Estate work. I considered my utility practice as a public service balance to the professional profit motive of my practice.

I looked upon my Friday evening TV program as a chance to relax before enjoying the weekend. Since 1989 I was no longer commuting to Hartford. I had become general council to the Cooperative. I was allowed the time to carry on an outside practice for two days each week.My commute was to Norwich a half hour drive.My position at the Cooperative also meant in ten years I would have a fully vested retirement pension with a defined benefit plan.

With the warming weather of May my wife and I hoped to enjoy the weekend sun. My worries had been set aside. Anything that might suddenly affect my health was not in my thoughts

On this Friday, May 15,1992 seven months after my dad's 100th birthday, my health abruptly changed. As I tried to stand up at the end of the television program, my right side lacked muscle control and sensations. I had no muscle strength throughout my right side. The side had no ability to feel even a pin prick. My mind was clear.My eye sight seemed normal. My speech was audible.My knowledge about friends who had suffered a stroke was that they had lost consciousness and had been rushed to a hospital. I convinced myself that the cause of this sudden change was less serious. After a sound sleep I would awaken in the morning with my normal health. I dragged my right leg as I moved to my adjacent bedroom, climbed into my twin bed, and fell asleep. I had told no one of the sudden change in my condition.

The next morning the weakness and lack of feelings along my right side remained the same. I knew that I needed to telephone my internist. The day was Saturday. I reached the answering machine. I said into the device that avoids human contact " my condition is an emergency." After a brief period of time another physician called. He was on weekend duty. As we talked the physician realized that my voice was clear and my mind functioning. He told me to rest and to stay in bed. I should see my internist early Monday morning. If there was any change to give him a call.

My anxiety began to border on fear.I had no choice but to remain in bed. My right side was not functioning. My wife,Ruth, was as confused as I was. I telephoned a close friend using my left hand, a neurologist specialist at Mt. Sinai Hospital in New York. His advice was the same to remain in bed and to have my internist call him Monday morning after I had been examined. The year was 1992.

I spent the weekend in bed with my meals carried to me on a tray. I could eat soft foods and drink liquids.My only movement was to drag myself to the bathroom with Ruth's help.I placed my left hand on her shoulder. I took my one bath to reduce any body odor. Early Monday morning my wife drove me to the internist. After a thorough physical examination he called the neurologist. As they talked it became clear even to me that I had suffered a stroke. The decision was made to admit me to Mt. Sinai Hospital in New York to diagnose the cause. My internist advised me to be transported by ambulance. I decided to have a good friend drive me to the hospital. I called the neurologist at Mt. Sinai to discuss my not using an ambulance. He made the arrangements so that I could avoid the emergency room. I thought that I would spend only a short period being examined by medical specialists. I was wrong.

The next day I was driven to New York resting on a pillow. At Mt. Sinai a portable bed was rolled next to the car.I was rolled to the hospital check in area. There the needed paper work was completed. My condition and my blood type were written into a band attached to my wrist. I was X-rayed to avoid a bacteria illness being introduced into the intensive care unit. My portable bed, with straps to keep me immobile to avoid my rolling off, went up in the elevator. I was rolled by the attendant into a six bed intensive care neurology unit. On four of the beds were sick patients.

For the next week plus the memorial day weekend I underwent intensive examinations with technology. Time in a hospital between examinations or surgery without family or friends visiting is often spent under going the commotion of a hospital or in boredom and anxiety.

Since my memory remained normal I used my idle time to reach into my long term memory. I recalled how my father had practiced medicine. Bringing forward these memories I found was a better use of my idle time than staring at the ceiling and worrying about the present.

The memoirs to follow compares two eras of medicine separated by fifty years. I will compare the differences in the time spent with the patient between the two periods. Each approach made a meaningful contribution to my recovery. There is a need to combine the best medical treatment of both periods. Without modern technology or most pharmaceuticals, the need to treat the whole patient and not just the injury or illness was a necessity when my dad practiced medicine. That the same need exists today becomes clear during my partial recovery from a stroke.

My Dad's Birthday Party

My dad on November 2, 1991, 6 months before my stroke, celebrated his 100th birthday. The party was held in Farmington, Connecticut at an assisted living facility near my brother's home. Dad had been living there for a year in his own small apartment. My dad received any assistance that he might need. As he had never learned how to cook except to boil water, all his meals were provided. Dad's interpretation of living in the assisted living facility was that he was the resident physician to provide needed medical care till a local doctor arrived.

His birthday party filled the dining area with over 80 people. All knew my dad as former patients, as a friend, or as part of the family. When the chocolate ice cream birthday cake had been cut, dad stood up at the speakers table, surveyed the smiling faces, noticed who had a cane, and how patients and family were mixed at each table. He separated his lips and opened his mouth into an appreciative smile." I deeply regret that there are none of my contemporaries here to join us. Their spirits are with me as well as their friendship and wisdom. Most of all I miss Libby who you all knew and loved. As she aged she became even more beautiful. She was a charming hostess, capable of an off color joke. She made our home warm and a joy to visit. Away she played golf and swam. Till prep schools she assumed the care of our three children so that I could always be a doctor caring for each of you. I became your friend and advisor. Some of you had illnesses or injuries that needed the best surgical skills then available to survive. I hopefully provided such medical skills.

I will relate a few of the instances when we first met and determined the need for surgery. Before and after the operation we got to know each other. I used my surgical and recovery skills. You knew how or learned to collect your thoughts to help with your own recovery. If you have forgotten, I can quickly detail these encounters."

Dad told four stories dating back 50 years. After each story there were smiles, eyes of appreciation, and applause. His patients both respected him and joined with him in feeling the warmth of friendship. It made no difference to these former patients that he had retired 17 years previously and had lived eight months in Florida for 10 of the last 11 years. For the first time since my mother died there were tears in his eyes. He was the best doctor I knew and a remarkable man. I looked forward to a party of my friends and living colleagues on my 90th birthday. Since I have a mix of genes not just my dad's, I look forward to my 90th year.

Dad paused and sat down to eat his ice cream cake before continuing his talk. I reflected on my own career.

I had not followed my dad's career and practiced medicine. After a difficult time with college chemistry at Yale, dad and I agreed that the profession of law could provide me with the skills to perform a service for others and to earn a livelihood. I would still be training for a professional career. Like dad I had a dedicated work ethic. I had had a law office in Hartford, Connecticut as part of a partnership. My home was a shore side house in New London. My parents had wisely purchased after the 1938 hurricane.

After forty years of professional practice I felt the strain from the demands on my time and the care required to analyze and to protect my clients against risks. The legal documents were exceeding fifty pages to close large real estate transactions. This was before the computer took control of the legal profession and increased the pages that could be spun out by the software memory to in excess of one hundred. Each computer had an adopted version of the so called boiler plate. The initial argument as to whose computer would produce the working document was an opening advantage toward the final agreement.

My hair had thinned and turned gray and was becoming white.

I left the private practice of law to reduce the pressure and to be able to continue working on an indefinite time frame. In the fall of 1989 I became general counsel for a cooperative utility. I had done the original legal and lobbying work that had established the Cooperative.The Coop provided electric power for five Connecticut municipalities. I was now a specialist as are most physicians. I was beginning to enjoy this different area of the law as I mastered the new words and specialized knowledge required.

Each day at the Coop I sat at my desk, a large mahogany desk and working table combined. I had acquired it in the early days of my practice. My office was made attractive by two of my wife Ruth's landscape paintings on the walls.The desk was covered with documents setting out the terms for the buying and selling of electricity. I read the documents with my glasses placed toward the middle of the desk. My pencil with heavy lead markings would check and then underline each area that required revised wording.My review would be checked by the engineer and the Director before being returned to me for the final wording. The language was unique to the operation of a utility. I knew lawyers in other areas of practice who would first need to learn the meaning of the words used.

When Dad finished his desert he again stood up unassisted. I quickly stopped thinking about my daily legal work. I was at the table with my dad enjoying each moment.The guests were also my friends. I had no advance knowledge of what Dad intended to say.

Dad focused his eyes behind his steel rim glasses. He faced the two younger physicians that he had encouraged to study medicine and who were practicing medicine in their selected specialties. He rambled on " Medicine today has changed. There are limits imposed by insurance carriers on your time with the patient. Both of you have become specialists. You limit your daily practice to your own specialty. It gives an old man like me respect for the explosion of knowledge in medicine since I retired.

During our medical careers I and my colleagues used the best medical skills then available. We had to know and to treat the whole patient. I had to spend time with my patients as I examined and helped them to recover. I learned about their symptoms and complaints. I knew enough so that they became whole people not just patients with a medical injury or disease. Only then could I, my patient, and the family join together to help the recovery. With good care and with my insistence on cleanliness, the body's own natural ability to heal helped to overcome many of the injuries or diseases with the aid of aspirin, rest, and liquids. A doctor pulled it all together and helped the patient to develop the will to recover. I loved the work that I performed every day. I succeeded without much technology or drugs. I had no choice. They did not exist. The patient's attitude was a key to the recovery. No insurance carrier told me that I was spending more time with a patients than they thought appropriate. Fifty years ago medicine was different. I've talked enough. I am getting tired. I am enjoying the party. I am delighted with the many who are here as survivors. I need to sit down like the rest of you."

My clinical study

Fifty years ago and prior to the many subsequent scientific discoveries, the whole patient was the key to the recovery. A physician spent more time with a patient. He listened to the patients complaints and observed their symptoms. He soon understood the patient's feelings and attitudes. He examined the patient with few tools of technology. He used his eyes, ears, nose, and fingers. He became a respected friend of the patient and of the family. He made available the needed time. Because of the time limitations imposed by the insurance payers for today's medicine and the reliance on technologies and pharmaceuticals, treating the whole patient rather than the disease or injury is not always integrated into current medical practice.

My one person clinical study of my exposures to these two eras of medical practice separated by 50 years will bring this message home.

My life had been divided between my profession as a lawyer protecting my clients, my time with my family, and involvement with public service.

My wife, Ruth, and I had enjoyed the vicissitudes of life..Ruth was a stay at home artist,. She was helped by my love of family during evenings, on weekends, and on vacations as we raised our four children. Otherwise she was on her own.

My wife and I had enjoyed each child in different ways as they matured and became adults. Three had left home. The oldest, Philip was a utility lawyer with a Boston law firm. He lived in Lexington. He had the same work ethic as my father and myself. My son Albert, a ceramic artist, lived in Japan. He inherited my wife's creative artistic talents. He studied with a master ceramic artist in Japan. He married a lovely Japanese woman after permission from the oldest member of her family, her grandmother.. Each son had one daughter. Albert's second child and our third grandchild, a grandson, was born four days after my stroke. The best news for me before entering the hospital. Our oldest daughter was in Washington with her husband, a nuclear engineer, and their pug dog, Otis. The youngest daughter, Anna, became mentally ill with a diagnosis of a by-polar disorder at age 18 while away at college.She was now living at a non profit out patient care program located in Vermont dedicated to bringing about the best sustainable recovery. Adjusting to her disability was my first intimate exposure to the malfunctioning of a person's brain.

My routine was to arrive at my home, a gray shingled wooden house close to the Sound, as early as I could. Despite this motivation I often did not eat dinner until after seven o'clock. Before dinner there was a need to break away from the work ethic and relax. My wife and I would drink a short martini as we sat on the out side open porch facing Long Island Sound. We could smell the salt air. If there was a wind we could hear the breaking of the waves. Dinner was often New England style cooking that could sit in hot pans until we entered the kitchen. As the days lengthened each year during the spring, the mood would improve. When June arrived, I would enjoy a routine of early morning swimming as the Sound warmed. The roof sky lights would provide more light. With commissions to paint landscapes, Ruth could sketch and work with oils.

The marriage had lasted through periods of harmony and of divergence. Our academic and childhood backgrounds were reflected in different interests. My background and training made me believe in the need to organize and to work toward achievable goals even when the goals seemed beyond my reach. Ruth focused on the details of the daily family life raising four children, shopping, care, discipline and encouraging their achievements. Her relief was to retire to the attic and to create an oil painting.We came together as a family on weekends and vacations. We both enjoyed swimming and holidays in south Mexico. I would play a tough game to win in tennis with her brother and a good friend Joe, a writer and thinker with Robert Hutchin's Fund for the Republic. Hutchin was the former President of the University of Chicago and had established the liberal Foundation. I kept the budget and made out the checks as Ruth had little interest in mathematics.

The most difficult period was the adjustment to mental illness. We had to work through the hereditary genes, the chemicals that affect the brain, and the growing up pains that changed a latent condition of our youngest daughter into a breakdown. No family can pass into such a changed environment without difficulty. We were no exception.

With our daughter beginning to enjoy a degree of recovery in the calming atmosphere of Vermont, we could again plan a summer trip to the cottage in Maine. The cottage brought forth Ruth's fond memories of her father as an artist and her summer vacations during her childhood. Gentle mountain climbs, popovers at Jordan Pond, and trips to isolated off shore islands filled my thoughts. There was the mix of a sense of the flow of the pleasures of life. The planning for the trip to Mt. Desert produced an atmosphere of climbing small mountains, picking wild blueberries, and relaxation without any thoughts of the limitations that age might bring.

The stroke was an abrupt change to the immediate future. After the stroke I spent the weekend in bed. I was hospitalized for ten days at Mt. Sinai Hospital I underwent numerous examinations by specialists with their technology. I have had a slow, uneven, and lengthy attempt at a recovery.

My initial decision to remain at home struggling with my condition is not an appropriate response. The correct decision, if you or your family have any awareness that the medical difficulty may be a stroke, is to dial 911 and go to the nearest hospital.

After the stroke,
Memories from my childhood

Even though I grew up in a medical family I had not kept abreast of the changes that had taken place in the practice of medicine. I lacked knowledge about modern medicine. The attempts to diagnose the cause of my stroke, the slow recovery, and my adjustments to permanent disability exposed me to modern specialized medical practice.

After my stroke, I had no knowledge of the damage that had occurred or the nature of the recovery that lay ahead. I knew enough to expect technology and drugs to be key catalysts. My mind, rather than remain in idleness and worry, recalled the memories that I retained about how my dad had practiced medicine. The pulling out of these old memories began as I remained bed bound the weekend after the stroke. The memory recall continued during the many idle hours at Mt. Sinai Hospital. When I returned home I added information gained from research and interviews.

In the attempt to diagnosis my medical condition at Mt. Sinai Hospital, the physicians tried to determine the cause of the blood clot that injured certain brain cells. The skills of not one doctor but many specialists were involved : neurologists, internists, cardiologist, hematologist, and physical therapists to help in restoring the lost muscle strength. Thirteen months after my stroke and removed from the need for any emergency treatment, the noted neurologist, Dr. Louis Caplan, duplicated my dad's approach..He spent the time to review both my symptoms and the technology pictures. He approached me as a whole patient.His examination was not just to determine the injuries suffered and the probable causes. He used the extra time spent with me together with the time of his younger colleague to become more familiar with me as a functioning person. His many previous patients allowed him to narrow his focus to my individual difficulties. He expressed in words that I understood what was and was not the cause of my hard joints and spasm.He added to the specialty of neurology, behavioral medicine. I began a new phase in my recovery. I developed the positive attitude to maximize my recovery.

The battle to recover became my battle to fight and to win each and every day. Without his explanation I might not have succeeded in accepting the limitations to my normal physical movements and the continual discomfort. The knowledge that I gained ended my depression.

My adjustments to the post stroke changes took years not days. There were serious set backs. It was over a year and my visit with Dr. Caplan before my emotions accepted that my stroke was not life threatening. There would be a daily struggle, but I could still enjoy my life. I had to change some of my planned retirement activities and to accept an earlier retirement. I would never play tennis or golf again.

My memories of my dad as a doctor were an invaluable resource. When they were combined with an understandable explanation of the affects from the damaged brain tissues, I had the emotional strength to reorganize my memory and to develop a positive control of my emotions. I could accept and no longer feel remorse about my condition. I could undertake the daily struggle. The right joints that felt in continual spasms and hardness were not damaged by the stroke. The damage was only to brain cells.

The human brain is a complicated organ. It controls the body, determines responses and emotions, and organizes memory into thoughts and action. Within the brain there are sections. The brain stores long and short term memory.The brain controls your muscle and senses of feel.The brain draws on instinct, logic, and emotions. The brain is the human being's interpreter. The nerves act as a message system. When brain cells are damaged by a stroke, lack of control and false signals can have their own reality. In my case the spasm and hardness of the right joints that I continually feel are real for me even though they are caused by damaged brain cells. The continual sensations would not be felt if these cells had not been damaged. When my nerve message system rejuvenated and became reattached to the damaged thalamus cells after eight months, the damage cells caused the adverse sensations. Until then, these after affects were not felt.

My memoirs interpret two eras of medicine. They provides a one patient clinical study of the importance of the whole patient. The frustrations that many patients feel about the limited time a physician spends with each patient did not take place 50 years ago. Patients exposed to the practice of specialized medicine need their GP as a medical quarter back to call the signals, explain each specialist's role, and to challenge the time limits imposed by insurance company payers. The medical practice 50 years ago was based on a close and warm relationship between the physician and the patient. The time spent by the doctor to explain to and to be understood by the patient made up for the more limited scientific medical knowledge. The patient could detail and describe their symptoms to the physician.

The earlier era of medical practice when I was a youngster became a beacon of light to help me to participate in my recovery. I recalled how my dad explained in ordinary words so that his patients understood their medical problems. My recalled memories gave me a new insight about my dad as a doctor. The imposed idleness and the motivation to remember pulled out of my memory all the details that were retained. They had not been part of the conscious every day use of my mind. It had been a long time since I had thought about how my father practiced medicine.

In dad's era of medicine there was a greater need to rely on the patient's own ability to recover. There were more frustrations because of the limitations of medical knowledge and the lack of discovery of most pharmaceuticals.

My accounts from this earlier period of medicine will reveal the need to involve the patient as an integral and key factor in the recovery. They also retell a warm and close personal relationship between the physician and the patient when the doctor was a physician, advisor, and friend. These are memories that very few possess today. They need to become part of the known historical record about the practice of medicine.

During the periods of idleness I once again became aware of the attitudes and methods of practice of my dad, a doctor between 1918 to 1983.

My dad's attitude toward each patient emphasized the importance of a doctor allocating enough time to treat both the disease or injury and the patient as a human being with developed attitudes and emotions. My dad medical practice is a fascinating tale revealed in the details of his treatments of and attitudes toward the patient.

Medicine Fifty Years Ago
Practiced by My Dad

In the spring of 1938, I went on house calls with my Dad. I was 10 years old. That particular Saturday I remember my dad,Dr. David Sussler, cranked the starter on his green Reo coupe and placed his black medical bag behind the seat. He motioned for me to settle in beside him and off we went to call on patients in Norwich, Connecticut, a textile manufacturing town of 38,000. He was a broad-shouldered man 6 feet tall with the physical strength that reflected athletic activities. His eyes were blue green behind his steel rim glasses.They penetrated as he focused on you during his conversations.

I remember him behind the wheel, confidently shifting the gears. His glasses settled onto his strong extended nose under his felt hat. His appearance conveyed a sense of his knowledge and empathy to which patients responded. Yet I only knew that he was my dad, the doctor, and that I liked him.

He was unusually talkative on this sojourn. His first stop was to a new patient. While he was not sure of what illness he would find, he did know how he would conduct his examination. As we drove toward the house, instead of whistling or engaging in small talk, he began a lengthy monologue. " I was old enough now to understand what the nature of his work truly was. A doctor must learn the details of a patient's illness on his first examination. He must get inside the patient by asking questions and most important, by listening to the answers."

"I will first ask this new patient about what I call his symptoms. Where does it hurt? The answers may make me want to know more about his past illnesses or injuries, and those of his family. I will ask about his life style. I will want to know what work he does. When did he feel ill, and why did he want to see me." This was a doctor's approach to medicine in 1938.

I sank down in the seat and began to look uninterested. He nudged me and added, "But that is just the beginning. As we talk, I'll go through the checklist any good doctor goes through. I'll notice the color of his eyes, face, and tongue, and his smell. I will use instruments, but the most important tools are my hands, my eyes, my ears,and my nose as I smell the odor and observe my patient. I'll feel his pulse and I'll listen to his breathing and to his heartbeat. My instruments are the stethoscope to hear any chest congestion, a flat stick to look at his throat, and the thermometer to take his temperature. By the end of the visit, I'll know a lot and the patient will feel better. Our encounter will have been just as much a discussion as a physical examination. If I can, I'll tell him the name of his illness so that his concerns can be reduced by the knowledge that I have had previous exposure to his medical problem. It will take nearly an hour" and he said smiling as I gave him a horrified look " I've brought the funnies for you to read while I work."

"But I will know what to do with this patient," he said, getting serious again. "If I am not sure, I will consult my medical journals. I might anyway just to improve on the diagnosis. I have additional tools of surgery and X-ray. If the disease is life-threatening, I will act quickly."

My father was as good as his word. His house call took just under an hour. He emerged with his patient, a boy twice my age, and one of the boy's parents. The diagnosis was appendicitis. We all drove to the William. W. Backus Hospital so that the boy could be operated on before the organ ruptured. My father's response was to drive to the hospital as it was quicker than calling and waiting for an ambulance. He was at the patient's home.

This was my first lesson in a physician's approach to medicine and dad's close contact with his patient. The medical lecture would be repeated to me again and again over time.

My father was proud to be a doctor. He knew that the practice of medicine was more art than science. Doctors like my dad used their medical skills rooted in their experience, their knowledge of the body's ability to heal, and judgments made with less scientific insight than now exists. The crux of his work was a balance of scientific knowledge, insight, and the personal empathy that he was so gifted in establishing with patients. Dad spent enough time with his patient to create such a relationship.

As a result of my stroke, I became a reluctant participant rather than a youthful observer of the relationship between specialists and their patient. I learned that the doctor patient inter exchanges that my father felt was a necessary part of his medical care were bypassed in the emergency conditions to try to find out the cause or causes of my stroke. Today, technology, pharmaceuticals, and economic efficiency have taken control of the modern practice of medicine.They form the parameters of modern medicine. There is the advantage of a vast increase of knowledge about the human body and how it functions. On the negative side, medicine today is subject to the cost controls and time limitations established by the insurance companies or the government agency that are the payers for medical service. There is the limitations caused because specialists are unwilling to discuss or treat medical problem outside of their specialty.

My stroke ended my 40 year career as a lawyer. I had to reorganize my memory and to redirect the use of my time. The morning after my stroke without my realizing it the changes began. My mind was not being used to organize details to win an argument or to produce a document ; instead, my brain recalled the experiences and attitude of my dad as a physician in a town of 38,000. When I had suddenly become unable to move about except with difficulty, I knew that staring at the walls or ceilings would add to my discomfort. I instead used my mind and memory to pass the time recalling my dad's medical practice. During my active professional days or during weekends and vacations with my family, I had not spent any time recalling this oral history embedded in my memory. The recalls were both a challenge and a constructive first step toward my hoped for recovery. I remembered his dedication to his patients practicing his medical skills.

My father's attitude as a doctor was rooted in his belief that he combined his professional training with a dedication to use his medical knowledge to bring the best treatment to each patient. He was not a perfectionist, but he believed that each person should perform to the best of his or her ability. That work ethic was intertwined with his moral fiber. A good doctor brought relief to his patients. His reward was the gratitude that his patients felt in return. If the illness lasted for any period of time, dad's doctor-patient relationship evolved into one of friendship. He spent enough time with the patient so that a friendship could come about. Dad knew that a doctor had an important role in helping the patient to fight the illness and in advising the patient and family how to adjust to any changes in the previous life style.

Physicians are now specialists. They lack the time to have the contact with the patient and the family. Specialized medicine today limits the physician to his selected specialty. His contact with the patient focuses on the treatment required within that specialty. Modern medicine especially at times of emergency care fails to involve the whole patient. The physician is not able to spend enough time with the patient. A patient may not understand the medical procedures that the internist and the needed specialists have determined are required to restore health. Doctors use technology rather than time with the patient to learn about the condition of the patient's physical body. The specialist then uses his or her skills to restore health and to fight the disease or malfunction with the aid of pharmaceuticals, radiology, or other tools of modern medicine.

My physical damage came about from damaged brain tissues. When I left Mt. Sinai hospital I lacked the energy even to return to limited professional activities, With the new imposed idle time, I began to read anatomy books and articles about the brain and strokes. I learned my stroke was caused by a blockage in the blood flow to certain tissues in my brain. For one week I lost full muscle control and the sense of feel along my entire right side. I learned that because I am left handed, the stroke did not affect my speech. The stroke had caused me emotional concerns but I did not cross the line to fright as I knew nothing of the risks and dangers, the consequences of a stroke, its causes, or the injury that a stroke could cause to one's brain and how that injury could affect the body. I have learned enough since to be a lay neurologist, but I am self-taught. I had none of this knowledge when I left the hospital.

There are two usual types of stroke. One type of stroke (ischemic) is when the blood flow to the brain is reduced or stopped by a blockage within the arteries or the smaller capillaries that must constantly bring blood to the brain cells. This flow of blood results from the heart's pumping that brings oxygen and nutrients to cells throughout the body. 25% of the body's blood goes to the brain. Without this constant flow of blood to all of the brain cells, the affected cells are damaged or destroyed. This blockage and damage is defined medically as an ischemic stroke.

The other type of stroke is caused by hemorrhaging. This occurs when an artery that brings blood to the brain from the heart, or a vein that returns blood to the heart, or vessels within the brain burst causing an uncontrolled blood flow that destroys brain cells.

I had suffered an ischemic stroke.

In an indescribable short period of time my right side had no muscle coordination. Without muscle control there was limited ability to move my right arm and right leg. I lost my sense of feel. A pin prick of the right foot or right hand produced no pain. My right facial muscles were immobile.

Because of my lack of understanding for the sudden change, I had faith in a full recovery. I could not believe or accept that I would spend my days confined to a bed or chair. I was convinced without any medical basis that my weakened and not normal condition was temporary. After all a broken arm heals in a matter of weeks. My dad had instilled in me the faith that an injured body can recover over time. I was unwilling to recall his patients that became permanently disabled. I had not known any of his patients who had had permanent damage to the brain.

Seven hundred thousand people in the United States suffer from a stroke each year and face an exposure to damaged brain tissues. I hope my clinical study of recovering enough to live with my disability when combined with my recall of the importance of the patient in medical practice 50 years earlier will help others stroke suffers and their families to understand the patient's and the family's role in the recover. The physician should devote enough time to treat the whole patient not just the injury or disease.

When I arrived at Mt. Sinai Hospital I had little understanding of the ramifications of the world that I was about to enter. I had so rarely needed medical treatment throughout my life that I might as well have emerged from a time capsule buried in the 1930s. All that I understood about the world of medicine I had learned from my knowledge about my father, a home-town family doctor, and surgical specialist who practiced in Norwich, CT., from 1918 until his retirement in 1973.

My understanding of this earlier period of medicine included my long term memories about my dad, a series of recorded responses made by my father as he reflected on his medical practice, discussions with physicians who had practiced with and learned from my dad,and the remembrances of a few of his surviving patients.

I will relate descriptive details of my father's practice of medicine during the 1930s and 1940s and earlier. They reveal the more limited tools that a doctor then possessed. They point out the existence of the close patient-doctor relationship. A doctor knew that he needed to activate the patient's own healing powers, the patient's psychological capability to cope, and the family's ability to help the patient. These were important curing aids. Doctors lacked modern medicine's technology capable of diagnosing the medical problem or the pharmaceuticals and technology that are able to improve or to restore health.

My father's world was one in which he made house calls on Saturday and many weekday afternoons. In his earlier years of practice in the 1920s before I was born, dad told me that he performed an operation on a patient's own kitchen table. Dad determined a medical diagnosis not from the use of MRI, CAT scans, ultrasounds, or a myriad of laboratory tests, but by talking with his patient until he had a thorough understanding of the symptoms and the circumstances in which they appeared. A patient's recovery was enhanced not by antibiotics, IVs, diagnostic hospital stays, treatment by medical specialists, or powerful new drugs. What was most important to the recovery process was the trust relationship between the doctor and patient. It was a trust that doctors understood would enhance the patient's own faith, willpower, and inner natural resources to bring about the healing necessary for recovery. Several of dad's patients, still surviving, have expressed to me the relief that they felt just by his entering their room. Dad knew that human beings usually survived because of the body's ability to fight bacteria or to protect the healthy portion of the body. He knew that the restoration of health needed the help of good food, liquids, rest, fresh air and will. His Yankee and Italian patients taught him that honey, garlic, and olive oil contained special ingredients to help the body's own ability to restore health. He used the medicine, aspirin, to lower the temperature. He also knew that success was not always assured.

This combination of self-healing and the early stages of scientific medicine were his curing alternative to the antibiotics that are credited with saving the lives of so many. Dad's early practice combined a belief in the art of medicine with the science of medicine. He began his practice in the twilight years before the science of medicine all but eclipsed the healing arts in which he so believed and which benefited his patients so much. He practiced the best medicine his profession could deliver from 1918 to 1973.

As dad's first lecture to me pointed out, the physical examination was an essential first step in treating a patient. Dad performed each physical examination as a matter of need. It not only brought a closer connection with the patient but also was the source of diagnostic knowledge about the patient's medical problem. The physical examination was an accurate diagnostic tool and much less expensive than modern day technology. The flat stick holding the tongue down to examine the throat could determine the motion of the roof of the mouth (stroke) or redness at the back of the throat (an infection). A look at the eyes under light revealed changes in the eye's blood vessels (high blood pressure) - or pressure from a tumor. Listening to the lungs could reveal one of the symptoms of pneumonia or bronchitis. The sound of the abdomen on the right could indicate a liver problem, on the left an enlarged spleen.Temperature could confirm the probability of a bacteria caused disease. Pain from thumb pressure on the right abdomen and a certain low level temperature were factors in determining appendicitis. During the examination the smell of the patient was an important diagnostic tool. The physical examination included feeling the pulse which revealed if the heartbeat was normal.. The physical examination by the physician should remain as the first diagnostic contact in the modern medical delivery system. The examination can allow for a discussion between the physician and the patient to reveal hidden symptoms and to prevent medical problems being missed. Diagnostic technology is most accurate if it is directed toward the cause of all symptoms which are affecting the health of the patient. Some symptoms may only be revealed after a thorough discussion with the patient. There are times when an underlying medical problem is not easy to detect except through a penetrating discussion with the patient. Modern technology without this knowledge may not focus on an undetected medical problem causing a delay before it is discovered.

Dad's training and early medical career are important historical anecdotes. My dad's attitude toward his medical practice and dedication to his patients reflects the attitude of physicians during this important period in the development of American medicine.I decided not to limit myself to writing down this earlier medical history as related to my stroke recovery. I will also deviate and write about unknown details of my dad's life and medical practice. He was the example that I knew among the many dedicated physicians who practiced medicine during the same time period. A life dedicated to medicine that needs to be recorded

At age 10 dad began to deliver the New Haven Register after school. He was able to supplement his mother's earnings from sewing and making dresses. His mother had been educated as a young woman by tutors in Russia together with one year studying in Paris. My dad's grandfather was a Jewish engineer and a member of the Russian middle class. They lived in Elizabethgrad, now part of the Ukraine. His grandfather had died two years before the entire family including his wife and their seven children emigrated to America in 1894.The oldest, dad's mother, was married with two children. After arriving in New York Dad's father managed a cigar store in Manhattan while the rest of the family moved to New Haven, Connecticut. Dad's father died after becoming ill with pneumonia when dad was 6 years old. His mother moved to New Haven to be near her family. Dad's young goal thereafter was to become a doctor and to help those who became ill. A deviation was his fondness for chocolate ice cream. As a paper delivery boy he had been allowed to scoop out ice cream as the proprietor of a confectionery store read the New Haven Register without buying the paper..

Dad graduated from Hillhouse High School in New Haven, Connecticut in 1910,He had excelled in scientific subjects. His goal was to attend Yale medical school and to become a doctor. My dad attended Fordham University where he took two years of pre-medical courses before entering Fordham University Medical School and graduating in 1916. He had wanted to attend Yale Medical School where his uncle had just graduated. But in 1910, Yale Medical School adopted a policy requiring four years of undergraduate training. My dad did not have the money to pay for four years of undergraduate studies..

From 1912 to 1916 my father was well trained at Fordham for a career in the medical profession. He studied the structures of the human biological system. Autopsies were performed on cadavers. Only limited clinical studies accompanied the academic program.His medical education taught him to scientifically analyze the human body but also to rely on the bodies own recuperative powers. There was emphasis on the need to provide the natural conditions for the body to restore its own health with rest, liquid intake, a balanced diet, exercise, and recuperation..Aspirin was the medicine to bring down a temperature. Doctors learned not only the importance of applying science to medicine but the limitations that then existed. The profession lacked the ability to cure many illnesses.Nevertheless there had been great progress. Medicine had repudiated blood letting and other procedures considered quackery. Surgery could remove diseased organs such as appendicitis, tonsils, or foreign bodies, and explore beneath the skin.

The curriculum at Fordham had been revised after 1910. Abraham Flexner after extensive research published his findings in a treatise entitled " Medical Education in the United States and Canada " The Carnegie Endowment distributed it to all medical schools. Fletcher pointed out the existing inadequacies in the teaching of medicine.He advocated and the institutions agreed that a standard curriculum was required. Clinical exposure should be incorporated into the curriculum. Dad 's medical instruction at Fordham Medical school used the new curriculum.. Fordham had adopted the Fletcher recommendations but was not inter connected with a teaching hospital.

Dad's course schedule at Fordham combined small classes with an excellent staff of teaching physicians. The subjects included anatomy, physiology, pathology, therapeutics, pharmacy, chemistry, medical jurisprudence, the theory and practice of medicine, surgery, obstetrics,and diseases of women and children.

On September 2, 1922 dad married the charming, well educated daughter of a wealthy Jewish family in Norwich, Connecticut. Dad took a year away from practice to study medicine in Vienna,Austria. His new wife my mother, Libby's, parents paid for the trip and studies as their honeymoon gift. In the early 1920s this medical center was more advanced than those in the United Sates in teaching scientific medicine. The medical school in Vienna taught that a physician had to learn how to investigate to determine the disease or injury causing the medical problem, to think scientifically, and to keep abreast of new medical information. The Vienna medical school taught dad to continue his medical training during his entire medical career. He learned the necessity of spending time with the patient.

My dad even with his surgical military skills and the advanced training in Vienna began his medical practice with the more limited scientific knowledge and training than available. He was equipped with knowledge and respect for a patient's own recuperative powers. He was well trained both academically and clinically for his era with the available skills and most important the attitude to restore health and to save lives.The patient was central to his diagnostic skills.

Equally important in molding the medical students mind were courses that were not taught in 1912 to 1916.There were no courses in the economics of office management or computer codes to appease insurance carriers. The many new courses now taught because of the increased use of technology and drugs were not part of the curriculum in 1912 as they had not yet been discovered.

During 1917 the country was hotly debating whether or not to enter World War 1. Dad wanted to be ready to enter the Army medical corps if the United States declared war. When he read an advertisement in the American Medical Journal of an opening for an intern at William W. Backus Hospital in Norwich, Connecticut, a textile center of 38,000, dad was not willing to pass up a career opportunity near his home in New Haven. Dad contacted the superintendent of the hospital, Mr. Hutchins. He agreed that dad could be one of two young doctors who would receive a $25 payment and would have a 6 month period of training as an intern. Dad would be continuing his medical education with clinical studies.

During his internship, Dad became friendly with Dr. H. George Thompson who was on the staff of the hospital. Dr. Thompson wanted to spend the summer at his cottage in Maine. He hired Dad as an associate to cover his practice while he was away. Dad had volunteered to serve in the army medical section if the United States declared war. There was an added agreement that Dad would be free to leave if called up for military service..

Dr. Thompson had begun to practice medicine in Norwich at the end of the nineteenth century. Many of his patients were mill hands who labored in the textile mills located in the Taftville section of Norwich. Others were members of the elite, the mill owners and the managers who ran the great brick edifices which dominated the riverbanks of New England early in the 19th century and beyond.

Dad practiced in Norwich for a brief nine months before being called to active duty. Dad was sent to the University of Pennsylvania Medical School for training in removing bullets and shrapnel and the surgical repairing of wounds. He was then sent overseas where he was attached to a British unit fighting with the French army at Ypres. Dad served as a medical officer in the trenches of France. When it rained his feet were covered with mud. German shells passed over his head until a gas shell landed too close and he succumbed to the gas.

He was transferred to England and the Estate of Lady Astor to recuperate. He rejoined his unit as it returned by troop ship to New York in the spring of 1919. He was discharged on June 3, 1919. He brought home with him a carved cane marked with the words " Argonne 1914 - 1916 " given to him by a French officer who had recovered from shrapnel wounds with dad as his doctor at a front line hospital.

Dad contacted Dr. Thompson in Norwich on July 19, 1919 and told him he was ready to rejoin his practice. Dr. Thompson told Dad he was his new partner, and dad began his long career in Norwich. In 1920 he became one of the first Jewish doctors to join the staff of a non-profit Protestant established hospital. The appointment to Wm. W. Backus hospital, the only hospital in Norwich, was arranged by Dr. Thompson who was then chief of the medical staff and doctor to some of the hospital's wealthiest contributors. If dad had not been appointed to the staff of Backus hospital, he was required to add the services of a member of the staff if his patient was hospitalized. This meant a splitting of fees and the possible loss of the patient to the staff doctor.

William W. Backus Hospital was starting to modernize its facilities but to my father's way of thinking, it still had a long way to go. Dad was a force for the highest standards of cleanliness and care. Dad specialized in performing surgery. The hospital had an ordinary sink at which doctors prepared themselves for surgery. They were handed a little scrub brush and soap, and they were told to scrub their hands for 10 minutes. Dad found a medical supply company that would provide disposable rubber gloves.

Sutures for surgery caused concern. In those days doctors took turns boiling their own sutures for surgery. My father was appalled. He deliberately spoiled a batch of suture material one day by boiling them so long they were unusable. Then he told the hospital to write to medical companies that were just beginning to sell ready made sutures for surgery. Hospital officials ordered the sutures. Doctors were freed from making their own sutures.

Dad insisted on another innovation. He required nurses assisting in the operating room to count all sponges and gauze used in surgery and to make sure the same number had been removed before closing the surgical penetration of the body. Dr. George Gildersleeve, then head of the surgical staff, made sure that these innovations improving the hospital standards were adopted.

Cleanliness within a hospital and cleanliness by physicians continues to be a medical problem. A survey by The Center for Disease Control and Prevention estimated that there are 20,000 hospitalized deaths a year of patients infected because doctors did not properly wash their hands as they made hospital rounds. It further estimates that 1.5 million patients a year will pick up an infection while in a hospital.

Dad's normal surgeries reflected the era in which he practiced. The most common surgeries in my dad's period of practice were for tonsillectomies, hernias and appendicitis. There also was the need for exploratory surgery as physicians were without the technology to inspect the body's inner structure except by X-ray. A doctor administered an anesthetic by putting drops of ether on a mask that went over the front of the face.

Surgery was dangerous in the 1920s and 30s because of the lack of antibiotics, but my father was accustomed to improvising from his service in the military. In a day when 90,000 people a year died from an attack of appendicitis, Dad performed surgery for infected appendixes with a new twist. He put a drain in the open incision, the better to contain infection. His patients chances of recovery improved.

In dad's era, doctors understood that bacteria caused diseases were contagious and were a danger to the healthy as well as the sick. Dad was aware that other family members could be exposed. He recommended that the sick person be kept in a separate bedroom and that family members not place their heads near the sick person's head when meeting his or her needs. He separated their utensils,dishes, and bed linens. In this time period there were no dish washers. Plates and utensils had to be washed by pouring boiling water over them.

Dad's surgical skills were used before all patients would accept the need to go to a hospital. One day he went to the town of Canterbury to treat a woman with tuberculosis. On the way back to Norwich, Dad ended up getting lost on the back roads and wound up hitting a boulder in the dirt road and driving his car into a ditch. A nearby farmer, named Bodin, came out with a pair of oxen, hitched them to his car, and pulled the car out of the ditch. Dad asked, "Bodin, How much do I owe you?" Bodin replied, "All you owe me, Doctor, is a promise. If my wife or I get sick, and I call, will you come to see me?," "By all means," Dad said.

Later, Dad recalled, "In the summer of 1924 Bodin called. His wife did not feel well. Dad drove his Reo car on the dirt roads leading to the farm house.When he knocked and Bodin opened the door,dad walked through with his black medicine bag. The house was a small wooden dwelling. The windows were divided into small sections to allow in light which revealed the interior wooden floors. There was a large long table in the kitchen for family meals. Bodin's wife was no bigger than five feet tall and weighed only 80-90 pounds. She was In the bedroom of their farmhouse lying on her bed. She showed dad her breast. It was all decayed from cancer. " Dad told her and her husband that he had to operate on her at the hospital. She replied, "I will not go to the hospital." Mr. Bodin said, "Could you do it in the house?" Dad thought about it and said, "Yes, I think I can. Youth has its advantages. You can not turn down a dare when you are young." Dad asked an operating room nurse from the hospital and the nurse in his office to help. He operated on Mrs. Bodin on the kitchen table and did a resection of her breast. He was careful to cut away healthy tissue around the tumor. " I had to do what I could to avoid missing the cancerous cells. I think I charged them $100 for the surgery. Mrs. Bodin made a full recovery and died at the age of 85 from pneumonia." Dad had given in to Mrs. Bodin fear of a hospital. He used his surgical skills without the protection of the back up capabilities of a hospital. He admitted quietly at a later time that this operation was the last time he knowingly compromised medical standards.

When Dad started his practice he was not a specialist and performed whatever medical services that were needed. He delivered babies at home for $5. Women called the hospital. They would send out a doctor to the address. The hospital would give the physician who was available a medical bag with the necessary obstetrical equipment. Dad would arrive at each home with a serious and caring expression. Years later he would recall the spiritual satisfaction that he hoped the family felt as a new life and the center of attention opened his or her mouth to begin the journey of life. One day, my father went out on a delivery without checking the bag. He said, "When I got to the house there were very few furnishings, just a bed and a table and a couple of chairs. No curtains. When I opened up the bag, it had just a few instruments, hardly any. It lacked tape, or a cord, or sutures. The woman had an uneventful delivery. When I looked for a piece of string to tie the cord off, they did not have any string. The only string they had was the one hanging from the shade on the window. But they did not even possess a pair of scissors. A friend of hers went to her house and came back with a pair of scissors, tailor's scissors, big long things. I cut the string from the shade and had it boiled before I used it to tie the cord off. Everything went smoothly but the incident stayed with me." Before dad left the home, he urged the nursing of the baby and lectured on the importance of cleanliness.

Before 1915 most doctors received their medical knowledge from their studies in medical school and during internships.Their clinical knowledge was from dissecting cadavers and occasional visits to a hospital during their internship. After they began practice they learned from older doctors who had gained knowledge from their experience.

As specialties did not exist, doctors served in a rotation covering all kinds of medical cases. Most doctors served in hospitals but they also served in free clinics, called dispensaries. My Dad said, "Dispensaries were for the people who were unable to pay the fees that doctors requested. The fees were very, very low, but still many people could not afford them. They went to dispensaries. The dispensaries had only one fee anywhere from 10 cents to 20 cents paid to a woman who recorded your name and address and gave you a doctor when he was free from treating other patients. You gave him your complaints and he would examine you and give you a prescription. It was more often a statement of medical advice than a drug to be brought in the pharmacy. In some of those dispensaries, they also gave you the medicine for free and told you how to take the medicine that the doctor ordered. In that way, medicine went along. You'd be surprised. There was a waiting list of doctors wanting to do this work. This work filled the gap caused by limited clinical studies at medical schools until the schools became part of teaching hospitals. Doctors were very willing and honored to dispense knowledge and care for people who needed to have the care, and yet were unable to pay any kind of fee. A doctor needed such experience, combined with his scientific training, to make judgments independent of technology.

Doctors such as my dad made medical judgments based on confidence and sheer guts derived from experience and education.

Because the best doctors had the affection and trust of their patients, these judgments, even if wrong, were not exposed to the fear of liability. There were few, if any, malpractice suits against doctors.

Dad had skills from his surgical experiences learned while in the British trenches. These skills increased the number of surgical cases in his early practice and led him to specialize in surgery during his medical career. He had the ability to learn just through observation. Once he had witnessed a type of surgery, or removed a diseased or damaged part from a patient, he knew exactly how to perform the same surgery on others. He improved his surgical techniques by accompanying patients who sought the expertise of the best surgeons practicing in the northeastern United States. He watched or assisted operations performed on his patients by Dr. Harry Cushing, the famous neurosurgeon, Dr. Robert Greenouph, and Dr. Lincoln Darin, at Massachusetts General Hospital in Boston. His photographic memory allowed him to duplicate these clinical experiences.

Equipped with surgical skills, he could remove a tumor, an infected appendix, and sew up a hernia. Dad could reconnect the digestive tract. He did exploratory surgery but only when he felt that it was necessary to discover the problem. In every surgery because of the danger of infection, he demanded total sterilization. He developed the innovation to drain fluids after an operation to avoid infections. In all his surgical operations, dad first conducted his own physical examination of the patient. He combined the specialty of surgery with the close patient relationship often now confined to a general practitioner.

Dad, during the first 20 years of his practice, fought disease caused by bacteria with few tools beyond aspirin, vitamins, liquids to prevent dehydration, a balanced diet, personal hygiene, exercise and the ability to activate a patient's will to survive, using the body's own defense systems. Cuts were kept clean with mercurochrome or iodine. Aspirin allowed a patient to perspire during the night as the disease reached a crisis and then subsided and the healing process began, Dad began the practice of medicine before most drugs had been discovered by the pharmaceutical industry together with their healing capabilities..

Dad knew that 80% of those who became ill would recover. The physician's role was to make the patient more comfortable and to speed the recovery. The physician gave the patient the needed sympathy and reinsurance. When the patient recovered, doctors faded away, and focused their skills on the medical problem of a new patient. The other 20% who became ill or injured required treatment by a doctor as essential to the recovery. Some would never fully recover. These per cent statistics remain as true today as when dad practiced.

Dad was confident of his own ability but he understood the dangers to which a patient was exposed before the 1940's revolutionary change in medicine with the discovery and use of penicillin. Despite the fact that he was an accomplished surgeon, he would often say that there were too many unnecessary operations. Before the '40s, he worried about the danger of infection. Afterwards with the availability of the bacteria-killing drug, penicillin, he worried about unnecessary surgery because of the new sense of safety. With the use of such drugs, Dad, and other surgeons, felt much more at ease using surgical skills.

Dad felt his limitations as medical surgery made the transition from the removal of pathological matter (organs, tissue and foreign matter) to restoration or replacement, the surgical refitting of the body and its organs. He admired the surgical skills in transplant operations and heart surgery, but he knew they were beyond his reach. His age was against him.

Dad performed many operations to remove an infected appendix. Many were young teenagers.A parent would call for Dad to come to their apartment or house.He would examine the young patient. He could ask both the child and the parent when the stomach area began to hurt. Where did the pain begin ? Where did it now hurt ? He would take the temperature. He would press hard against the lower right abdomen and let go. Was there an out cry from pain. He would make a judgment if there could be a collection of mucus in the appendix. The temperature level would help him rule out a bacteria caused stomach pain. Was there vomiting or diarrhea ? All these details came from the young child and his parents with dad at a home examination. A diagnosis of appendicitis required quick surgery before a rupture. The child needed both parents and doctor's reassurance to reduce fear. The needed surgery in the hospital meant a scary experience. Dad knew that the pain following surgery was related to the skill in the surgical cut and removal of the appendix.

His success at being paid was another matter. Dad himself admitted, "I did not care about money." During most of my father's medical practice, there was no insurance carrier to make payments. He often did five operations at the hospital during the 1930s and was paid for only one.

"I'll never forget the Depression," my dad recalled. "I operated on a woman in 1932 whose family name was Gilman. She and her husband had been married for some time. I operated on her and removed an acute appendix. It was not ruptured. I dissected it out and she got better. This was during the Depression of the 1930s. I sent Mr. Gilman the bill for $50. He came into the office and said, "I appreciate the amount of your bill. I consider that very nice of you. I felt like it would be much more. But I can not pay you. All I get is $800 a year." I said, "Mr. Gilman, how do you get by then?" He said, "I bake pies and sell them to people who go to my church. With the dollars I can make on pies, I can live." In 1936 he came in and paid me the $50. He said that the dividends from his stock holdings had started to come in."

During the Depression, as Dad said, "People got sick and went to the hospital just the same." During those years the hospital had a terrible time making ends meet. Dad suggested a plan. He discussed with the hospital that it institute a flat-rate plan. When a patient had a tonsillectomy, the hospital would charge $15. The hospital got half; the doctor got half. That way the hospital could get some money until the economy improved. Hospitals suffered because charitable contributions were in an abyss caused by the depression.

Dad took care of the poor including many immigrant families without pay. Whether he was paid or not for his medical services did not influence the way he carried on his practice. Finances were not part of his medical training. This attitude was borne out by his patients. Proof of that occurred every Thanksgiving.

Every Thanksgiving, Henry Lucas brought a turkey to our house. And every year, as my father cut into the bird, he told the story. Mr. Lucas' daughter had a serious malfunction, a blockage of the intestines. The doctors, who had examined her, felt there was nothing they could do. A friend had suggested Dr. Sussler as a final hope. Henry Lucas had little money but told Dad if his daughter survived that he would provide a turkey every Thanksgiving. Dad operated, removed a section of the intestine and restored the health of his daughter. He had seen the operation done once, in Boston, in the early twenties when Dr. David Jones, professor of surgery at Harvard Medical School and chief of surgery at the Massachusetts General Hospital, had operated on a patient of Dad's for a similar problem. Henry Lucas' daughter had symptoms that included diarrhea. Dad had previously arranged for Dr. Jones to do exploratory surgery on an earlier patient with similar symptoms, Crosby Grover, the son of the manager of the Ponemah Mills textile factory. Once Jones had opened the area he remarked, " I have never seen anything like this before." There was an inflammation of the small intestine near the appendix. Dr. Jones removed the section and then he reconnected the intestines, the process of anastomosis. My father was able to duplicate the procedures used by Dr. Jones and save Mr. Lucas' daughter's life. In the process, he provided for us a turkey every Thanksgiving.

A physician today does not have the time to accompany a patient undergoing surgery to a large teaching hospital to watch an operation being performed by an internationally famous surgeon.

Dad had a great respect for teaching hospitals as medical centers. This was especially true of Massachusetts General Hospital in Boston. In 1939, my older brother, Frank, became ill from a streptococcus infection picked up while swimming in the pool at Phillips Academy Andover, the prep school he was attending. Dad thanked Andover when he learned that my brother had been immediately transferred to Massachusetts General Hospital from the Andover infirmary. At the teaching hospital, they were not only able to have the curing skills of the best surgeons as Frank's illness required removal of the bone in the forehead to drain the infection. The hospital was aware of the drug sulfonamidine as a result of the British discovery of sulfa drugs in 1938. With the use of this drug, they were able to stop the bacteria from multiplying. My dad knew that without this drug and the available surgical skills, his son would have died. The success of the medical care that my brother received resulted in his being still alive. Teaching hospitals continue to provide the medical profession with the training, professional skills, and research for improving medical care.

In my father's era doctors spent many hours with over extended work days, applying their skills for the benefit of their patients. The schedule dad maintained throughout his professional career speaks for itself. His day began at 7 A.M. After a breakfast of toast, juice, and milk, he would drive the ten minutes it took him to arrive at the hospital.His operations began before 8 o'clock and continued until he had finished the three or four or the one if very complicated that had been scheduled. He followed surgery with hospital rounds visiting patients who were recovering from surgery. He would return home for a quick lunch. He would then spend a forty five minute period relaxing with friends in a card game in a confectionery store across the street from his office. His office hours were from two to four PM. He would devote a minimum of 30 minutes to each patient. He returned every weekday evening for office hours from 7 to 8:30 PM.

After his afternoon office hours he would visit patients at their homes until his arrival at our house just before 6 for dinner. His schedule for Saturday morning was to make house calls in Norwich and the surrounding towns where his patients lived.The time it took him to complete these calls depended on how long he thought the patient and the family needed his presence. This included his curative skills, psychological reinsurance, or the time the family needed to learn how to be helpful in aiding the patient to recover or to adjust. He responded to each patient's call including those who he knew were hypochondriacs.Requests for appointments occurred within days. He felt it was unresponsive to delay a patient for weeks or months. He understood how important the early detection of a disease or malfunction could be. Emergency calls were received on his three digit telephone that could interrupt his activities at any time including Sunday, the one day that he spent with family or friends. Vacations were not part of his schedule. Yet he suffered no burn out. He loved medicine.

A mark difference in how doctors were paid for their services existed. During the 1920s, a medical colleague practicing in Sprague, a nearby mill town, called Dad because of his wartime experience to help on a case. A 6-year-old boy had, on a dare, tried to jump over the skylight on the roof of a movie theater. He did not make it to the other side. The boy crashed through the window and hit the floor below. The boy's own doctor did not think he could be saved, and asked Dad to look at him. The child was comatose, with multiple fractures, including fractures of the frontal portion of the skull.

Dad put the boy in his car with his father holding him, drove him to the hospital..After the anesthesia, Dad repaired the skull as best he could, irrigated the area, and sutured the skin and tissue. After Dad set the last fracture, he knew the healing process was up to his young patient, who did not have the benefits of antibiotics. Penicillin was invented two decades later. Dad hired nurses for round-the-clock care to take care of any emergencies. Because the boy's family had no money, dad received no payment for his medical skills. Dad paid the $100 cost of hiring the nurses. Fortunately, the patient recovered and was out of the hospital in two weeks. In today's world of insurance payments, the situation for a doctor to do this may not occur.

Fees were straightforward. In 1916, when my father interned at Wm. W. Backus Hospital, most people hospitalized were assigned a bed in a ward. The beds cost a dollar and a quarter a day. Those who had enough money paid for a private room which cost three dollars a day. Doctors who visited patients in private rooms charged a fee. The hospital did not allow physicians to charge ward patients a fee.

My dad practiced private medicine for those who could afford to pay and would not charge those who could not. There were dispensaries to give free out patient care and ward beds in hospitals for the poor. Both supported by charitable contributions or free services.

Dad had a one man private practice. Doctors were usually sole practitioners. Two or more surgeons would join together to assist each other in complicated surgery. Dad earned $750.00 a week in the 1940s. He believed as an accomplished surgeon he was earning a high income for a town the size of Norwich.

Dad's billing system for his medical services involved his nurse looking at the charts of each patient being treated and with Dad's input determining the charge for each visit as well as any surgery performed. His nurse spent two hours a week billing patients. If the bill was not paid, it remained dormant. Dad was convinced that he gave such good medical care that the only possible reason for non-payment was when the patient had no money. There were no insurance coverage, no HMOs, no computers or computer codes and little paper work.

The only deviation from this billing procedure occurred when Dad needed money to pay for my brother's lengthy hospitalization. All the other medical care from physicians treating my brother was free. The practice between physicians was to give each other, and their families, reciprocal health care at no cost. There was the need to pay for the hospitalization of my brother, and my mom's stay in Boston to be near him. My mother insisted that Dad secure the services of a patient who was a bill collector. He reluctantly agreed. In a month and a half, enough money was collected to pay for my brother's hospital bills and the other debts.

Today, a physician's billings bypasses the patient. After the completion of the complicated paper reports and computer codes the bills go directly to the insurance companies involved. Patients are expected to have private or government medical insurance. Insurance did not begin to cover the patient population until after the 1940s. Only doctors who have elected to practice outside of the Medicare system bill directly to elderly patients with the expectation that the patient will pay. Private insurance normally covers the patients under 65 except for the uninsured. Physicians still can have uncollected bills for their medical services to the 43 million or more Americans who are uninsured. Physicians now accept a determination of the appropriate fee for approved services established by the insurance providers.

The economic rewards from the practice of medicine were not the motivation that kept dad dedicated to his medical practice. It was rather the self esteem from the use of his skills to maximize each patient's ability to recover even with the more limited tools that were then available. Dad's clinical experience developed in the trenches of France and in his practice and an uncanny ability to remember and departmentalize gave him an unusual ability to recognize quickly from a patient's symptoms the disease or injury. Dad was able to make a quick and accurate diagnosis of the medical problem. His medical care would include helping the patient to adjust to the probable outcome. Dad discussed at the appropriate time the health plateau that the medical symptoms might leave behind. This required time devoted to lengthy conversations with the patient. He would name the illness, address the cause, and was willing to predict the probable outcomes after weighing and addressing the odds and the patient's emotional ability to make the adjustment. He viewed his practice of medicine as patient-oriented.

My father judged each patient's ability to cope with an explanation of the probable course of recovery. He would be truthful but would use soothing language to help the patient understand the alternatives. He would make a judgment about the patient's ability to adjust to the new health plateau. Dad felt that a patient's understanding was a necessary ingredient in the curative process. He had the ability to restore confidence as he mixed his medical knowledge with the art of conveying a belief in the healing process. He would say, "a good doctor treats the disease, a great doctor treats the patient."

He understood that the family living at home with the patient also had a key role in the recovery process. They are in a better position to ask the tough questions that the patient who is unwell or medicated may not be able to do. The family needs to understand the details of the illness or injury so that they have an intelligent sympathy about the suffering and the adjustment that the patient's medical problem is causing. They need to understand the proper balance between time with the patient and time when the patient needs to rest and be undisturbed. They need to be made aware that many patients will have moments of irritability. Others, isolated from normal activities, are inclined to monologue at length about their limited knowledge of their medical condition. In today's practice of medicine, the doctor usually does not have the time to involve the family with an explanation of what to expect and how to help.My family had little knowledge of what might occur during my recovery, an unfortunate omission as my case history will illustrate.

Dad's approach to his patients was clearly expressed by another physician who was able to publish his ideas in medical journals, Dr. Lawrence Henderson of Harvard Medical School. Dr. Henderson spoke a language that Dad felt gave a more academic tone to what he felt. Doctors needed to approach each patient as a social being and not as another medical case. Today this attitude toward the practice of medicine would fit the term *social pathology*. Good medicine requires an empathy with the patient.

When my father stopped to examine each patient, his manner made the patient believe that his concern was wholeheartedly and exclusively focused on the patient's welfare. He would sit next to the patient's bed. After feeling the pulse and looking into the throat with a stick or their eyes with a narrow flashlight, dad would quietly ask for an explanation of where was the pain ? Did he or she have trouble with their bowls. If it was a first visit when did the patient feel sick.? He would listen to the patient's responses.If the answer was long winded and deviating from the information required he would redirect the conversation. The patient knew he had my dad's undivided attention..As he formed medical judgments he would discuss these with the patient. If more time was needed to make a diagnosis, he promised an early response.

His judgments, without today's technology, were rooted in his scientific approach, intuition and experience, and self-confidence in himself, as a doctor. This combination was reflected in his demeanor which showed no sign of arrogance. His warm humane approach required longer visitations than spent by today's specialist, but it resulted in both respect and trust from the patient. Often during this period of medicine with limited pharmaceutical breakthroughs, the doctor knew the recovery process depended on the patient's own self healing. His advice about family support played an important role. The body has a natural healing chemistry that functions to restore and to maintain a state of equilibrium. In many recoveries the body's organs achieve enough repair to perform their essential life continuing role even though there is not a full recovery. To accomplish this there must be a commitment to recovery within the patient.

I remember dad returned home after his Saturday house visits. I was in my mid teens. A look at his eyes that lacked their normal sparkle and the frown face told me something was wrong. To help him avoid keeping it all within I asked him what was wrong ? He was silent in thought for a moment then looked at me for understanding. " I went to see a long time patient. He suffers from limited muscle control. I restored his self esteem and he tries to act normal when he can. Just before I arrived he had dropped one of their wedge wood china dishes and it broke. As I entered the house his wife was screaming and trashing him for an accident that he could not prevent except by giving in to his physical limitations.

When she saw me she could not stop the flow of bad language. I stayed and sat on the kitchen chair until it stopped. I explained his difficulty once again. I told everyone that his need to try to act in a normal manner was essential for his attitude and health. I left with a sense of achievement until as I reached the door the angry flow of words started. These are the frustrations in bringing the best care to my patients that become deep disappointments. I learn that not everyone listens to me.A doctor's role is limited. I unfortunately know this but it makes me sad."

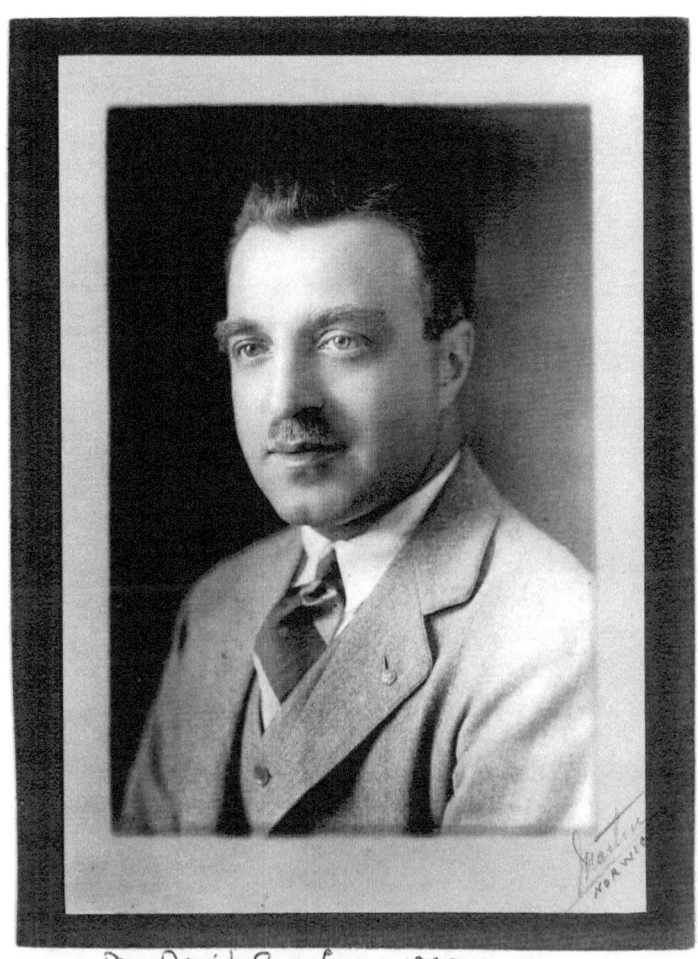

Dr. David Sussler - 1928

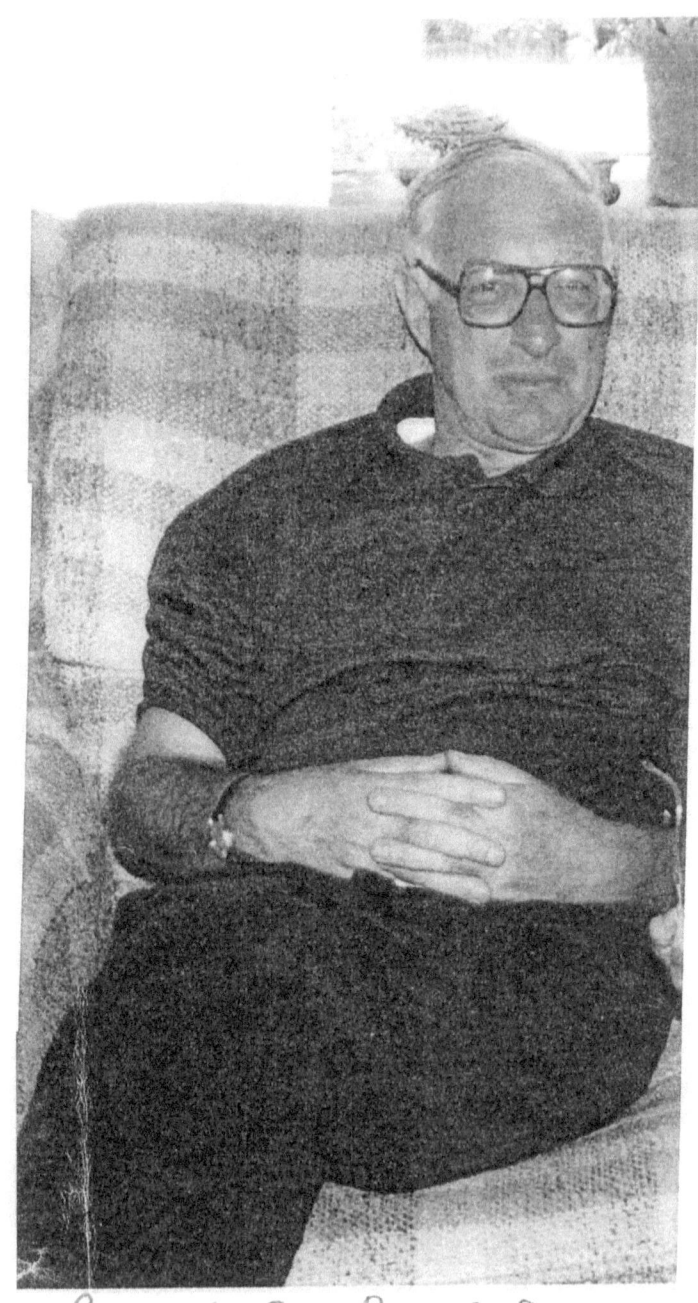

Robert Sussler 1998

Patients Reflect on My Dad

Dad's patients recalled him as a doctor who was a respected friend. As Buddy Grant said, "a classy guy." Interviews with patients now very elderly confirmed that he was more than the family doctor. For many of his patients, he was not only a skilled doctor but he was also the best available interpreter of the American culture. Many patients were immigrants lacking any formal American education. Dad was often the most educated man they knew. He combined his medical knowledge with advice on how immigrants could cope with their adjustment problems in a new culture. He was a trusted and wise figure in the lives of many; and not only for those who had recently come to this country.

Dad's patients have a vivid recall of their medical experiences. They focus on his attitude and approach, and on the limited medical resources that were available. Interviews with men and women in their eighties with good memories provide detailed anecdotes, an aging oral history that confirms my own memories from childhood. They all referred to my father as David or Dr. David, a verbal reflection of the sense of trust, respect, and understanding that he achieved with his patients.

As Chuck Savage remembers, Dr. David would come to his house, as he was the family doctor. " He made house calls as each of us (there were 4 children) succumbed to the childhood diseases of mumps, measles, scarlet fever and chicken pox. When he would come into the house after a couple of sniffs, he would tell our parents which one of the diseases one of us had. Then confirm his smell diagnosis by a careful inspection. His first smell proved to be a correct naming of the disease.

My father knew that an illness affected the body's temperature. He knew that the blood flow pumped by the heart to bring oxygen and nutrients and to remove waste could be affected. He knew the affect an illness could have on digestion and bowl movements. These were changes that altered the smell of a patient. Dad knew that the smell test could help identify the illness.

Chuck remembered that he was always gentle. " If I had a fever he would prescribe some type of pill. I guess aspirin. " What young Chuck liked most was that he would recommend that it be taken with Canada Club ginger ale. As Chuck recalled " A treat for me to drink something other than milk or water. I can remember the sympathetic expression on his face. I never sensed a need on his part to rush his visit. He would hang around after the examination and talk to my mother and father."

"There was one serious injury. My father worked in a coal yard. One day he got tangled in the machine that lifted the coal. They carried him home dirty and he was mangled. They placed him on his bed and called Dr. David. He came quickly."

"First thing he told my mother was to get the kids out of the room. He took a look at my father and decided he should not move. There was a man named, Haughton, who had just acquired a portable x-ray machine. He called him to come right over and he took some x-rays. It was early in 1928 or 1929. There was no cast necessary but David had to tie some splints. One was to stop movement of his thigh. My father was in bed for 3-4 weeks. Nature took its course and he recovered. David stopped by every second or third day."

"There was another night when my father decided we needed David as soon as he could come. It was about 1932. I had a belly ache all day. Toward evening, it got worse. David came over. It was for him an emergency call. He felt my stomach. He took my temperature and pulse. He looked at me. He told my mom and dad, I suffered an acute appendicitis and he had to operate. I was scared. He took me to the hospital in his car and calmed me down on the way. He had called the hospital from my house. When we arrived, they took me into the surgery room. My memory stops when they applied ether. Even though

David kept saying everything would be all right, I was still scared. I stayed in the hospital 8 to 10 days. When I was in the hospital, Dr. David visited me twice a day. He always sat in the chair next to me. When it was time to be discharged, he drove me home. About 2 weeks later I developed a blood clot in a vessel located in the area of my lung. David's face looked concerned. He had me lie flat on my back and told my parents to permit no movement. He knew it had to dissolve itself with no drugs to help. I got better so I guess it did. I remember my father, Jake, asking for the bill to pay for the surgery and care. David did not have a bill but said $100 would do. My mother took the dollars out of a draw and handed the money to Dr. David. It was more money than I had ever seen. "

By the forties medical specialties were beginning to be a necessary part of the medical delivery system. Medical knowledge of the human body rapidly increased requiring new specialized medical skills. As Chuck recalled " Your dad made his patients aware that one reason that they could trust him was his willingness to involve a specialist early on. Many doctors still waited before recognizing the limits of their skills. When Chuck Savage's father had pains in the urinary tract, your dad sent him to see his friend, Dr. Demming at Yale Medical School. Dr. Demming diagnosed that Jake had a cancer of the kidney. Your dad and I drove to New Haven and watched the operation. On the way back to Norwich, your dad described to me every detail of the surgery. Your father assumed I would be interested in learning the same details that interested him as a doctor. "

My dad's patients looked to him as a medical resource whenever they ran into a problem that they thought had a medical solution. In 1942 Chuck wanted to enlist to be part of the war effort. The recruiters in New Haven, Connecticut rejected him when they discovered a hernia during the physical. Rejected and dejected he called my dad. Dad said to meet him at the Backus hospital at 5 p.m. He alerted the surgical department. By six he had fixed the hernia. Chuck said, "I spent 2 weeks in the hospital and fully recovered. Your dad stopped in each day on his hospital rounds. On discharge I asked your dad for a bill. He smiled. Until they accept you in the military service, we do not know if we were successful. Your dad even gave me some cosmetic covering to hide the scar. I passed the induction physical. He never sent me a bill."

One day in 1929, when my dad was out of town for the day, Chuck jumped down from a tree in his back yard, a rusty nail went through his foot. This was late June. Chuck's father was able to reach my dad by phone at his beach house in Niantic. Dad told him to take Chuck to a Dr. Brophy at his home on Prospect St. When Chuck and his father, Jake, arrived they found Dr. Brophy smoking a cigar and having a sip of brandy. He looked at Chuck's foot with the rusty nail protruding. He pulled out the nail and jammed the opening with gauze, wrapped around a stick, covered with iodine. "Did I scream!" It did not bleed much. I went home bandaged. As this happened in the early forties and before the normal use of the tetanus vaccine, Chuck was lucky. Your dad came a day or two later. The area around the wound was purple. It was infected. Your dad told my father to buy leeches at the nearby Drug store and let them suck out the pus. We did it for a few days. It was less colored and sore; but still there was an infection. Next we tried salted pork. And the salt ocean water. They worked.

"My aunt, Charlotte Allen, saw your dad in the 40s. She had an aneurysm, weakness in the blood vessel wall. Any increase in blood pressure was going to burst the artery and it would be curtains. Your dad sent her to Leahy Clinic in Boston. They suggested surgery. With low odds for success, she refused. A week or two later, your dad was reading a medical journal and read that they were doing research on lowering a person's blood pressure with new drugs at Mt. Sinai in New York. He sent her to see a young doctor, who had studied medicine after your dad had told his father that it was the right profession for his son. At Mt. Sinai, they were able to lower her blood pressure with the new drugs and save her life. She was able to go back to work. Your dad was always reading the latest medical journals. "

His patients' families would call on your dad to decide family problems, to restore harmony after an argument, to determine a child's education, and to select a profession for their child. When your dad could, he would make phone calls to help the youngster get accepted in the professional school. Your dad helped hundreds, hundreds. Right or wrong whatever he suggested was done. He could say no wrong. It usually worked out all right, a remarkable man."

Dad cared about more than the medical problems afflicting each patient. His home visits expanded his knowledge into a full understanding of each patient Jake was slowly transferring ownership of the lumber business to his son-in-law. Jake had come to Norwich as the youngest brother of my grandmother's large Jewish immigrant family. He was one of Norwich most successful businessmen.Dad was aware of the difficulties that occur in the changing attitudes between generations. The family had full trust in his fairness and accepted most of his recommendations. Jake and Buddy thereafter worked out their differences.

Chuck Savage knew dad since being a child. His parents had looked to Dad for advice on the education of their children. Dad was more than the attending physician. He was a friend and confident. When Chuck needed help to understand the occasional depressions suffered by his wife., Dad suggested that Chuck include his wife, Iva, in his business doing the bookkeeping to provide her with daily activities outside of the home and to give her an added position of need and importance. Most of her depressions were eliminated before the discovery of pharmaceutical antidepressant drugs by a format that kept her busy and created a feeling of self worth.

My Dad's Attitude

In place of the seven stages of life in Shakespeare's "As You Like It " Dad talked in terms of the plateaus of life caused either by a breakdown of one's health or age. He would spend time with a patient to help him or she accept the new plateau and the physical limitations. He understood that this help would relieve some of the difficulties during the psychological transition period and would help the patient to accept any pain or discomfort. He used understandable words drawn from his medical scientific knowledge and from his insight about patients derived from his years of experience. His aim was to motivate the patient into a positive attitude, to maximize daily activities, and to accept the new physical limitations. His words were designed to instill a positive thought pattern and to rearrange the patient's memory to accept the transition to a new health plateau. He knew that each patient had to avoid the pretense that no change had occurred. He believed there was no reason to fear and every need to accept the new health plateau. It was one of the necessities as you adjusted to the changing patterns of life. Dad believed these adjustments were helped by the will to survive together with rest and nourishment.His favorite illustration of the body's natural defense mechanism was the protective wall that contained the infection within a boil.Whether dad had read Shakespeare's Seven Stages of Life I never knew.

I recall dad explaining the importance to motivate a patient. A man and friend owned and ran a successful small business. He came down with pneumonia before penicillin. For many days he had a high fever and was in danger of death. He finally passed the crisis of the illness and slowly started to recover. He was very weak and unable to stand. He spoke in slow softened words about lacking the will to struggle. Dad assured him that over time he would return to work. His prior good physical condition allowed his body to draw on an accumulated reserve. Dad had his wife and oldest son tell him how much they needed him even if he should not have his previous health. With dad's help they motivated him to join in the fight to recover and to do it each and every day. His attitude change helped his recovery. Dad had treated the body to fight off the illness but also the patient to take on the struggle to recover. He returned to work part time in six weeks.

He recognized that the new health plateau involved a spiritual adjustment. He encouraged a patient's tendency to monologue with repetition about the physical change and what the patient thought were the roots of the condition. Dad look upon this temporary change in the patient's usual verbal discourse as the patient's own memorial service to the healthy existence that was becoming part of the past. Certain patients would concentrate and verbalize on observable physical details. Their sentences could become repetitive. Dad looked for and encouraged an inner strength to take hold with their spoken thoughts again reflecting the patient's logic. The patient's conversation would again reflect their normal conversational word flow. The body, he believed, had a built in chemistry for survival. Dad had observed that there was a greater chance to shorten the recovery period if the patient achieved a positive mental attitude.This attitude he knew would have an affect on the patient's daily activities both his physical movement and mental concentration. When the patient focused on each day's activities it aided the healing. It restored self esteem and as a by-product reduced pain. Dad looked upon this combination as the coming together of spiritual support with the physical healing. He knew each patients would achieve this combination with different degrees of success.

Dad knew that each patient was different. There were no generalities or scientific terms that he would use to cut short a visit. After he diagnosed an illness that he knew would be lengthy or lack a cure, dad spent extra time to learn details about the patient, not just the disease. He needed both the patient's confidence and trust. Without these ingredients in their relationship he would be less able to help the patient in coping.

Dad's patient physician relationship with the serious ill or permanently disabled began with his awareness of the needed psychological adjustment while the patient was in the hospital.He would repeat during each hospital visitation with the patient that their attitude will be important in improving their recovery. With the first visit at home he would bring the immediate family together with the patient to begin the emotional understanding that a part of the former healthy patient so vivid in their memory would be slow in being restored or had ceased to exist. Each one would have to accept the change. He told the family that it had similarities to a mourning ceremony. Each ritual had its own uniqueness. Each patient had different memories, different inner resources, different tolerance of discomfort. He or she would have to adjust their memories as they came to accept the ending of certain past activities that their current health would not allow. A most difficult adjustment took place when a patient had to adjust to continuing pain or discomfort. As pain was interpreted by the brain, he knew that less idleness and more concentration of the mind could lessen the discomfort and dad hoped lower the level of pain.He knew aspirin and the newer pain killers would help reduce the pain. Some patients accepted periods of suffering fortified with a spiritual acceptance from their religious background. Dad encouraged these thoughts but the relationship a patient had with his or her God he left to their spiritual clergy.

Dad's philosophy was more scientific. He thought in terms of a humanistic obligation to carry on a meaningful life on the new health plateau, even if more limited and uncertain.

Dad had me visit with him one Saturday morning a woman patient. She was lying on a bed in the living room. When we walked in she smiled. Dad introduced me. There was a board on her bed with a pen. She slowly picked up the pen and wrote for a long period. She handed me the paper. The writing was so small it was difficult to read. The words had allegories with nature interwoven into a poetic rhyme. I was impressed. She whispered that I should keep the poetry. When we left dad told me what I saw were symptoms of her illness. He told me how happy my visit had made her. Dad reached out to help his patient's attitude even when the illness was so devastating.

The shutting down of a patient's responses caused by exhaustion and the inability of the mind to have a logical thought pattern, made dad realize that he had become a separated bystander. If the condition of the patient improved and healing again took over, dad encouraged the family to join in stories with humor, tales of vacations and events with the children and grandchildren. He urged quiet listening when the patient was able to talk and the recording of what was said to create a sense of the patient's own posterity. The patient needed to reestablish his self esteem. These were dad's acquired wisdom. His memory contained each patient's individualized adjustment. Dad had acquired this knowledge over many years. He had made the conscious decision that his role went beyond scientific terms and medical descriptions, definitions, conclusions, medicines and medical treatment. He would cross the line into the patient as a whole being. He took the time to understand the individuality of each patient.

Dad's told me his greatest frustration was the limited ability to help the patient to fight cancer. He said that in the future science would find a cure but he feared that this would not occur until after his lifetime.

The most difficult role for a doctor and for a patient is the final chapter, a patient's acceptance of death. Dad understood this was a time when the organs and chemistry of the body lose their ability to function and life will soon sans everything. It was the only time in his patient relationship that dad felt his medical tools helpless to do their needed recuperative functions, except to reduce pain. There was to be no earthly future. It was a time when he had to watch the patient enter the final passage from a living existence. He felt it important to keep the patient as busy as their health permitted and to concentrate the mind on the immediate without the idleness to think ahead. The presence of family members, even if they remained silent, helped interrupt the boredom which would cause moments of fear. Dad had to await for a physical deterioration whether it be pneumonia or just the closing of the eyes into permanent sleep to bring the sadness to an end. The body was no longer strong enough to function. His medical training could no longer prevent death. It was the most difficult part of his practice as it is for all physicians. His last action was to hold the hand as the patient reached out for the last time. More often a loving family member made this last moment of contact. My dad walked out of the patient's room saddened. He had done his best. They had become friends. He had treated the whole patient not just the disease or injury.

When dad returned home and after a period of silent thought said to me "I did my best ', I knew his skills had not saved a human life. When the death happened during the attempt to remove a ruptured appendix from a young patient, he could not avoid an emotional connection with the young patient and the family who could no longer enjoying any hope for the patient's future. Dad could unwind and control his inner emotions only after a brief sharing with one of us, more often my older brother., The extra time dad had spent did have an emotional side affect.

Dad's commitment to the practice of medicine and his devotion to his patients required the extra time to learn the attitudes and knowledge of each patient and their family. How much did they know about the medical condition and the nature of the recovery ? He knew that he had both to listen and to speak in a plain language to overcome their ignorance of medicine I looked upon him as the best doctor I could know.

Medicine Today and Hospital Care

Modern medicine, when faced with the emergency conditions to discover the cause of my stroke, lacked the time to bring me into the specialists circle sharing their knowledge. I was a patient lacking understanding or an awareness of the scientific language.

My medical care after the stroke provided me with another personal experience and exposure to the practice of modern medicine. My post stroke medical experience revealed the changes that have taken place since the era when my father practiced medicine.

An important change is the use of pharmaceuticals now available to prevent diseases and injuries and to supplement the bodies own protective capabilities.

Due to pharmaceutical advances since my stroke, a person who suffers any type of stroke today should go to the emergency room and be hospitalized immediately. The blockage causing an ischemic stroke may be treatable with newly-developed drugs; TPA – tissue plasminogen activator, approved by the FDA in 1996. These drugs must be administered within three hours of the stroke. The blockage can be dissolved by these new drugs and prevent permanent damage to brain cells. It should only be used to treat an ischemic stroke when the patient is not already taking an anti-coagulant, according to the latest clinical studies. Their appropriateness can be determined by use of technology, an MRI and CAT scan. These technologies will determine if there is a danger of an aneurysm occurring.

I arrived at the hospital with no previous hospitalization or any exposure to modern medicine. This new hospital experience at first reminded me of when I was drafted into the army during the Korean War. At the hospital I had to fill out the paperwork, mostly medical insurance data, be x-rayed, be examined by a medical assistant, and given the standard uniform:, pajama bottoms, light blue, along with a smock that opened in the back. I had my name and medical data stamped on a bracelet. Men are segregated from women. Each are given a bed of the same size with their name and a summary of their medical condition and precise instructions attached to the front of the bed..

Patients are mere inductees distinguished only by disease or bodily malfunction. In a hospital, individuality becomes secondary. The medical system of hospitals are caste societies run by doctors who, if ranked, would be generals. Lower-ranking officers and sergeants are nurses and orderlies, respectively. They are not allowed to provide any service not included in their job description. The care they provide is usually performed with both efficiency and kindness. Except in the intensive care unit, they physically stay separated from the patient unless called or when adjusting apparatus or dispensing medicine.

The atmosphere of a hospital creates a mood where a patient loses his or her dignity and privacy. The atmosphere eliminates the patient's individuality. They become human organisms needing medical attention.. Patients become one community united with the single purpose of getting well enough to leave the hospital. Hospitals today are a type of modern factory with an automated as well as skilled medical delivery system.

A modern hospital is neither quiet nor hospitable. I spent hours in drafty corridors waiting for a machine to analyze me, or for an orderly to wheel me back to my room after a test. The hospital procedures were not to call for the transportation orderly until the test had been completed. The patient, for whom the hospital exists to help, often feels that he or she is treated as superfluous and unimportant except when his life is in danger or he or she is benefiting from medical skills.The patient is dehumanized by this impersonality and detachment.

If I managed a hospital I would begin by allowing individuals a choice in the color of the pajamas, greet those who are able to respond, and make an attempt to use an understandable vocabulary. Patients can be approached as equal in status with the members of the hierarchies within the institution. These changes would have no impact on cost or hospital efficiency.They would greatly improve patient morale.

The specialists, except when in the intensive care unit, spent limited time with me because they wanted to wait for the data from technology. There are also the dictates of insurance reimbursements with payment limitations controlling the time spent with a patient.

While in the intensive care unit the neurologist acted like my dad and visited me 3 times during my 24-hour stay. While I was in the intensive care unit, instruments performed constant monitoring of my blood pressure, breathing and heartbeat. The intensive care unit gave the medical team time to continually observe me. I had time for my brain to rest. When I was transferred to a four-patient bedroom, I joined the large group of hospital patients whose lives were not considered endangered but who had a medical problem requiring treatment at a hospital.

In the intensive care unit, I had various electronic attachments reading my blood pressure, heart beat and temperature.My nourishment was from an intravenous bottle above my bed. I was very quiet and confused by the rapid changes after I entered the hospital.In the intensive care unit I remained immovable on my back. When I turned my head to the left I saw two nurses sitting on chairs. To the right was another bed with a man looking much weaker than I felt. He was surrounded by family. My reaction was that he is much worse off than I. The night became quiet. Sleep took hold after I closed my eyes. There was no one who required me to utter words. I am not sure what the chart contained about my ability to talk. Whether it read that I was left handed and could talk I will never know.

After 24 hours in the intensive care unit I was wheeled into a room with 4 beds. Each one had a male patient on his back lying quietly. There was a telephone next to each bed. Each of the patients in the room were able to converse but all were silent except when they were talking to a nurse or to their specialist Emotionally I was in a state of dependency as if I was again a child. I knew that I would have unknown machines or readings with electric impulses producing electronic graphs as they examined me.The times of being wheeled on the mobile bed to these examination rooms were also the times that briefly ended my idleness. My meals were another change from the boredom. I was again eating and digesting food and liquids. These long periods of idleness increased my confusion and uncertainty. The idleness while in a hospital lowers the patient's self esteem. I regretted that I was alone in the hospital. The visitations by love ones are important because it reconnects with normal human warmth and activities even when the conversation is silence. Companionship rather then a flow of words gives a needed reassurance.I was helped as I focused on my dad's medical practice.

Specialists were in charge of my care supported by nurses and orderlies. Nurses took blood pressure, temperature, administered drugs or took blood samples. Nurses would respond to the patient with sympathy and kindness. Orderlies brought bed linen, warm water for washing, and bedpans as I was still bedridden. Volunteers brought meals. Other orderlies transported patients to the location of technology for diagnostic tests. The patients saw less of the physician specialists.

My life was no longer subject to any threat. The specialists waited for the data from technologies.The specialists made their rounds with more time between each visit. They needed to compare the many electronic pictures. During each visit a specialist stood over my bed for a period never exceeding more than 15 minutes to inform me about the technology being used within his specialty. During those visits I realized there was less need to find out information from the patient. My mind was active and the physicians knew that I was conversant even if ignorant of my medical difficulty. I was not included in the analysis of the diagnostic examinations that had to be occurring.

My father made it a habit, during his rounds, to sit in a chair next to the patient's bed as a non-verbal reassurance. He spent as much time listening as talking. In contrast during my hospitalization, each of my specialists – the cardiologist, the internist, the neurologists stood next to my bed and because of my limited awareness of my medical problem spoke in a monologue to explain the machine or technology that would examine me to aid him in making a diagnosis.

Reliance on technology to discover the cause of my stroke had replaced the lengthy conversations and detailed observations my father had conducted as a matter of course with each patient. The personal trusting relationship between doctor and patient considered so vital when my father practiced medicine had been drowned out by the whir and graphic results of machines and made redundant by the results of lab tests. Therefore it should not have been a surprise that not a single specialist would discuss with me the likely cause or damage from my stroke until computer analyzed results were available and reviewed.

Hospitals try to respond to the needs of the patient. The operation of a hospital is subject to the limitations imposed by the payers of the bills, the insurance carriers. Insurers challenge the length of stay at a hospital and the charges levied. They can determine if a procedure is medically necessary and reimbursable.These controls hold down the reimbursements. A hospital in addition needs to pay cost increases, medical care in the emergency rooms, and the many millions of dollars of capital costs to acquire new technologies. With empty beds the per patient costs increases. When there is a gap between revenues and expenses, hospitals depend on gifts and grants or the ability to borrow funds to pay these deficits.

Hospitals have become corporate entities run with budgets under the control of corporate executives trained in overseeing the management of the hospital including cost controls. As gaps occur in the annual budgets, hospitals depend on annual fund raising drives and the ability to borrow money. Grants are a source of funds especially for teaching and research centers.

The result is that hospitals are less comfortable than in my father's time.William W. Backus hospital had many private rooms where families could visit usually undisturbed.The patient in private rooms often had private nurses who watched their progress, reported difficulties, and were a source of human companionship.The costs were within a middle class budget. Ward patients, roomed with their many fellow patients, were under the watchful eye of nurses who could be seen from each bed.

Although there is limited patient physician contact, nurses unless specially trained, can not intervene to improvise on the treatment until prior physician approval.A fellow patient was suffering severe pain.The nurse knew from the chart that another type of stronger pain killer would be appropriate. She had to wait an hour to reach the doctor. The right to reach a medical supervisor with quick access to the information should be standard policy in all hospitals. If extreme pain occurs, there should be rapid approval for an alternative medication.

The manner in which a hospital functions disturbs a patient tranquillity and the need to rest. Commotion takes place as each patient receives their medication or other assistance. With 4 or 6 patients to a bedroom, the noise disturbs other patients. Sleep and periods of quiet are interrupted. These disturbances may not occur in smaller hospitals lacking patients to fill the empty beds.

When a patient is awake and able to function there is little done to provide entertainment except for the TV and the telephone. Boredom becomes a depressant.The patient feels isolated without normal communication and contact. The psychological by-product is anxiety. As patients often suffer from pain, patient's withdraw into themselves.

Hospitals are institutions that are under pressure from physicians and patients to be up to date with the latest technology.Even in small hospitals millions of dollars must be spent without regard to the amount of needed medical use that may thereafter occur. Physicians push to be able to use the technology. Local hospitals are pressured to keep up with large medical centers in their technology.

Some hospitals are attempting to reduce boredom. Art programs have been introduced when patients are well enough to participate. Voluntary readers quietly visit and read to a patient or to groups of patients.

Hospitals are being designed with more private rooms monitored to observe the patient from a central location and the technical instruments to record any changes in their condition. Constructed hospitals are too expensive to convert to single rooms.

Hospitals have imposed internal administrative procedures to limit their exposure to liability.Patients must sign waiver forms recognizing the dangers of the procedures. If there is time a hospital wants to perform the preliminary tests rather than rely on fax transfers from another institution.

Physicians control the hospital to bring a high degree of skill, technology use, and rapid performance. The remaining staff are subordinate and contact the physician for information and input in methods set up by physicians.The administrative structures reduce the time physicians spend on administrative duties not connected with their specialty skills.

Technology is the Modern Method used to Examine a Patient.

Technology has taken control of the medical care system. Each instrument provides the data for a physician's judgment. A medical decision is not made without the use of all the latest producers of data, analyzing each and every part of the body that are appropriate to an understanding of your medical problem. I succumbed to the process by agreeing to all of the recommended instruments of diagnosis. I was examined by a CAT scan (evaluates brain tissue), the magnetic resonance imagery (MRI) (creates a sharp image of the brain to show damaged cells if the area involved is large enough), electrocardiogram (EKG) (rhythm of the heart), electroencephalogram (EEG),(recording electric impulses from the brain), ultra sound (tests arteries), a microscopic device to examine the heart, a doppler test (speed of blood flow), dye contrast (flow of blood) and blood analysis for blood viscosity (thickness), blood cells and blood platelets (ability to clot). Gone is the need for exploratory surgery.

The euphemism of the word technology did not mean that all tests took place smoothly. When I was to start the test with a dye tracing the blood flow, I was asked if I was allergic to fish. I said "no". The injection followed.I soon had difficulty breathing. I complained loudly.An offset was injected. I was then asked if I wanted to proceed or try again. Since I was already part way I said "keep going". The test showed nothing abnormal.

Not once did I question the use of the technology or the risk I might be taking by avoiding any technological examination. I would be accepting the physician's opinion without the use of the technology.I gave thought to relying on the cardiologist's opinion as to whether my heart was functioning normally but I agreed to microscopic images from the tube down my throat. My weak condition stopped me from deviating from the physician specialist planned evaluation of probable causes. The cardiologist, a considerate physician, admitted that one or two of the tests had the added purpose to protect him against litigation in the event they showed a problem.The microscopic examination of my heart, he responded, had a 5% chance of revealing an undiscovered problem. As the insurance would pay I said nothing.The examination was negative.

By the conclusion of all the tests, my insurance carrier would receive hospital bills over $30,000. If I had taken the risks and avoided the uses of technology, myself, my family, and the physicians would have turned our backs on modern medicine, but it would have made no difference in my ultimate treatment and path to partial recovery. The medicine of fifty years ago would have achieved the same result. However, in many other stroke situations, the use of technology does make a difference, a difference that can save the patient's life.

The Specialist and the Patient

When I entered the hospital and became the subject of diagnostic investigation through the use of medical technology, I assumed doctors still looked upon a patient as a whole person, suffering from a disease or injury. I expected specialists to use technology as wonderful tools in a scientific approach, but at the same time they would involve the patient in an understanding of the process so that he or she was made aware of how they fitted into and was part of the recovery. I thought of them as professionals dedicated to helping the patient to understand and to become aware of his medical problem, enhancing his ability to come to terms with his new health plateau.

Medical specialists as I underwent my emergency medical treatment to find the cause of my stroke left me with the feeling that their need to investigate the cause was more important than lengthy conversations with me. They were interpreters of technology. They would determine from the use of technology whether or not surgery was required; or what drug might help within their specialty. During the visitations, specialists directed little focus toward me as a human being with normal anxieties. As each test was completed, a specialist would look at my chart and then pause, standing by my bedside. The physician would assure me that no findings of a problem had occurred within the focus of his specialty. When I asked "What next?" the specialist would generally put me off by saying when the tests were completed, the neurologist, who had pulled the team together, would poll their findings and make his recommendations.

Each patient roommate was having similar experiences. Each was hospitalized because of a different ailment. As the room was in the neurology section, each of us suffered from an injury or disease of the brain or nervous system. I had one uniqueness admired by my fellow patients. As I had a team of specialists and each of the other patients relied upon a single neurologist, I had many more visits with physicians. I was spending much more time with doctor-specialists. Unaware that my discussions were little more informative than those each had with their single specialist, several expressed envy.

The discomfort I felt from lack of muscle strength and the anxiety due to the uncertainty of what lay ahead made it difficult for me to watch TV, the one available form of entertainment. Nor could I concentrate enough to read. The hospital is a treatment, diagnostic and surgical center designed to move patients in and out as fast as sound medical treatment permits. In performing these functions hospitals are uncomfortable and noisy. They are institutionally limited in the ability to consider the affect that this atmosphere might have on a patient's self-esteem. The family has an important role in humanizing a hospital for the patient.

Despite the multitude of tests using all the most sophisticated technology available, the specialists were unable to determine the cause of the blood clot. There was no heart or liver problem. The arteries showed no unusual sign of plaque accumulation beyond accumulation caused by my age. My blood pressure was normal. Yet I had suffered a stroke and there had been at least temporary damage to cells within the brain and to adjacent nerve tissue. The damage had initially affected the muscles on the right side and the ability to transmit feeling from my right side.All controlled by the left side of the brain. A right handed person would have had speech difficulties. As I was left handed my speech control was on the opposite side or the right side of the brain. There was little speech interference. The loss of feeling and muscle control were the visible and appeared to be the residual affects of the stroke. This indicated at least temporary damage to cells within the left cerebellum portion of the brain.

While these diagnostic activities were going on, the hematologist continued to test for any abnormalities or deficiencies in my blood that might reveal the cause of the blockage.

I had now reached the end of the diagnostic role of technology. Because of the three day Memorial Day weekend, I had already been in the hospital longer than my insurance carrier thought appropriate. It was time for me to leave. As the insurance carrier held the purse strings, it exercised a high degree of control.

The neurologist in charge conferred with the other specialists without me. Their objective was to reach a consensus of the cause of the blood clot and my future treatment. My only exposure to understanding any injury and their causes would occur in the final one-to-one conference with the neurologist the night before discharge.

This last hospital visitation lasted five minutes longer than the others but was still limited to a discussion of conclusions. My times spent with my father during the late nineteen thirties as he made his hospital rounds left me confused by the lack of feedback solicited from me, the patient. I was also troubled by the limited knowledge I had acquired. Yet I was still physically too weak to force doctors to give me the details concerning how they made their judgments to relieve my uncertainty. I was not well enough to carry on a lengthy two way conversation.

The neurologist expressed his relief that technology had eliminated causes that might require additional medical treatment as each specialist had ruled out a medical problem caused by the organ or the part of the body to which he had limited his medical career. The neurologist assured me that nothing life threatening had occurred. His conclusion was that I should take a daily dose of two mg. of coumadin, a blood thinner. It prevents blood-clotting agents forming in the liver and a baby aspirin as an anti-coagulate to reduce the odds of another stroke. Aspirin inhibits blood platelets from sticking together. He told me to have my blood pro thrombin monitored weekly until it reached the desired level, then monthly thereafter. He warned me to avoid cutting myself. My questions about the residual affects of the stroke drew no clear response. The neurologist merely reiterated that the technology had picked up no evidence of permanent damage. There remained the unknown. Only time would tell if the stroke had caused permanent damage. I would need recuperative exercises to improve the strength of my right side, arm, and leg. The neurologist told me that the doctor in charge of physical therapy would visit with me the next morning to outline the needed program for improvement.

There was no give and take, no exchange between equals. I was too weak and confused to ask tough or detailed questions. In this last longer exchange between specialist and patient, I did not achieve an adequate analysis of my medical condition and the prognosis. Such a discussion would have needed a reach out into me to help me to understand the difference between damage to other parts of the body and damage to the brain. A discussion in language that I understood without using medical terminology.

There was little feed back from me of my knowledge about the implications of suffering a stroke. This lengthy period of patient discussion and involvement, which my father considered essential for a successful recovery, did not take place. The discussions with me covered the medical history deemed appropriate for a patient to know before being discharged from a hospital.

The neurologist was not certain of any residual damage and did not want me to create verbal corners that might require such a response. Even a calculated judgment concerning probabilities would have reached beyond the findings of the technology and involved the risk of his being proven wrong in the future. These were exposures that a modern specialist is often reluctant to take; but which my father felt necessary even if done with a euphemistic vocabulary.

Early the next morning, the physician in charge of physical therapy and his assistant appeared by my bedside. The brief examination included testing my muscle strength, sense of feeling, having me slowly walk the hallway, and testing my reflexes. The doctor then showed me exercises to strengthen my arm and leg. He gave me a pamphlet with diagrams on post stroke exercises. Finally he gave me his card so that my local therapist could call him should the need arrive. The examination completed and recommendations given, they left.

The nurse in charge of the room broke my idleness. After 10:30, the hospital would charge me for another day and my insurance would not pay. She said it was time to leave. As soon as my transportation for home arrived, a volunteer wheeled me to the hospital exit. I packed my toilet articles and was ready to go. The nurse handed me the neurologist's prescription for coumadin. I left the hospital. The chauffeured limousine took me to the home of my in-laws in Norwalk where my wife was waiting to drive me home to New London.

Belief in a Full Recovery

I had a strong faith in my ability to quickly recover.. After my discharge from the hospital and the return to my home, I focused on how many days or, at worst, weeks it would be before my energy level would be restored to normal. I would return to work when my muscle strength was restored and my brain was once again able to direct my muscles to perform their functions. The neurologist reinforced these positive feelings by his advice during my first office visit to keep my mind active and not to dwell on my current physical condition. He did offer a limited sense of the difficulties that might remain. He said that I should be able to fully function even if some numbness remained in my right fingers and toes extending to the hand and foot. I was not to become frightened at a sudden loss of energy. On such occasions I should move my feet up and down or change the angle of my body to change the blood flow. His final sentence was neutral. My recovery would be what it would be, but there would be setbacks as well as improvements. I had yet to understand that noticeable recovery would be a matter of months or years not the days or weeks that the normal recovery from injury, illness, or surgery takes. I had no forewarning that any serious set backs would occur.

My exposure to modern medicine left a respect for the medical technology available in 1992. Although it failed to pinpoint a cause for the blood clot, it was successful in eliminating in a few days the many factors that did not cause the stroke.

I learned that the reliance on sophisticated technology made specialists reluctant to make decisions prior to the results of each medical test or the cumulative readings from several tests.

Modern specialized medicine tends to be adverse to and void of an emotional bonding between the patient and the specialist. I felt a reluctance on the part of specialists to treat me during my hospital stay as having an equivalent intelligence level with an understanding of my medical difficulties. I had a lack of knowledge of medical terminology and the scientific underlying data. This separation affected my morale. Scientific diagnosis from the use of technology was accomplished with a high level of efficiency. It has become the focus and source of a specialist's medical judgments.

Physicians Today

After returning home I had idle time except for my physical therapy, eating meals, and the need to rest. I began to read books borrowed for me by Ruth from the library about medical education today. I had been an avid reader of materials that filled gaps in my knowledge. I began to research the training received by medical specialists. To learn more about medicine today, I read about the medical school courses that made physicians the specialists who were treating me. I wanted to have a general understanding of the role of medical specialists in coming together to determine my injuries. My hope was to avoid fears from the unknown I learned the difference between an ischemic stroke and one caused by hemorrhaging. The lay medical books I read contained limited information about the brains structure. I would later learn much more.

I wanted to understand the roots of the changes in the physician's attitude toward a patient in these two different eras of medicine. I knew about my father's medical training. I learned about the training today of doctors from medical school professors who are now teaching the subjects and material.

The current medical training of physicians teaches the medical student the vast new knowledge and information about the human body, the technical sophistication of the machinery, the new medical alternatives, and the reliance on drug treatment advancements. These advances had not yet occurred when dad went to medical school. Medical training today gravitates toward specialized medicine. Each specialist stays within the skills of his specialty. The result is less reliance on the whole patient with the body's own recuperative powers.

Medical schools today provide the basic courses under the same descriptive headings; but they include the explosion of knowledge about the human body since 1912. Cadavers are now graphic and computerized; drugs are broken down into families and compatibility; surgery utilizes microscopes, providing internal pictures with graphic feedback as to the exact location of the tissue or foreign matter being removed. Surgery makes use of robots.Medical training relies upon and emphasizes technology and pharmaceuticals. Medicine is approached as a science with the doctor's role to determine the appropriate drug most suitable for curing or prevention, the need for radiology, or surgery and how to use the available technology. Medical schools are connected to teaching hospitals so that clinical training is included.

There are many new requirements taught a medical student as he prepares for a medical career. Doctors must be made aware of their exposure to liability suits. They learn methods to increase their economic well being. The trained doctor is taught to be part of a team of specialists acting in unison. They are taught that a general practitioner can act as a bridge between the patient and specialists. The diagnostic role has shifted from experience and observable signs to reliance on technology. The medical profession depends on the use of computers, software and cellular phones. They are part of the medical system that alerts a doctor that an emergency exists. If these tools of the information age involving Internet technology fail to accurately function, there needs to be a perfected back up system such as superior trained nurses or a medical rotating oversight to quickly react to an emergency.

The explosion in medical knowledge includes the new scientific understanding of the functioning and composition of a human being. There is a vast new reservoir of medical knowledge. Numerous new courses are included in today's curriculum : molecular physiology, cell biology, pharmacology, microscopic surgery, laser or gamma surgery, chemotherapy. Specialization results in a focus on a particular medical problem not on the whole patient.

Medical school today costs more than $45,000 a year. The annual charges have changed radically. When my dad went to medical school he earned the money for the year ahead by working as a conductor on a streetcar in New York City each summer except one summer as the medical supervisor at a summer camp in Maine.

In both eras, physicians must have a dedication to their profession and are willing to accept the required work ethic. Even though specialists may no longer spend lengthy periods with an individual patient except for complicated surgeries or other difficult medical problems, many long hours of work still occur because of the total patient load, the amount of information and data to review, the limitation on compensation for many examinations, most noticeable the compensation for internal medicine, and the overload of paper work.

Today groups of doctors performing a single specialty, join together. Doctors can no longer afford to act as single practitioners. It is only through group practice that they can own the necessary technology, have the non-medical assistants to do the paper work, pay the high rents at the proper location, and have time away from their professional work load. Group practice has become a necessity. In cities, doctors have delegated the preliminary examination of a patient to a non-doctor medical assistant. The doctor can then quickly review the findings and reduce the time with the patient. By this efficient use of their time spending only minutes with the patient, they examine enough patients to make money despite the caps placed on each examination by insurance carriers and Medicare.

Physicians no longer take the patient's weight, blood pressure, heartbeat, and temperature, or if required, a urine specimen or a vial of blood. All these activities were part of my father's examination as he got to know the patient. Only in small towns with a limited number of patients may a physician do these tasks.

Physicians are still overloaded with work. Time is required to keep abreast of each new medical development and the recent FDA approved drugs. Paper processing has become time consuming even with extensive use of the computer.

Even with the limitations on fees established by Medicare and insurance companies, the earning capacity of a physician has greatly increased. Busy specialists earn between $150,000 and $500,000 per year or more. Those unusually skilled specialists, who are sought after, can charge above the limitations placed by the insurance carriers and reach a million dollars in annual income. Only general practitioners (GP's) and pediatricians have more limited incomes.Their income can average out to $65,000. Fewer physicians seek out a medical career as a general practitioner.

The physicians earnings are achieved even though liability insurance, which was non existence 50 years ago, now costs at least in the six figures. Dad told me there were no suits against doctors except in California.

The average person in 1950 paid $100 for his medical care each year. This is the equivalent of $500 in today's dollars.The physician charges 50 years ago were in line with the billings my father felt were appropriate for his medical services. There was a minimum of technical equipment and there was a lack of pharmaceuticals. Each was a factor in the low cost of medicine in 1950. However, life expectancy was 68 not 78.

Today medical costs average $8200 per person or a total of $ 2.4 trillion a year for health care. This change is partially caused by fees that reflect the physician's new awareness about the human body and the need for specialization, new expensive equipment, and the wide use of pharmaceuticals. The science of medicine has discovered that high cholesterol and high blood pressure can cause heart attacks. Expensive drugs can triumph over such diseases that in the past were fatal. These changes have been noted by David M. Cutler in a little book entitled "Your Money and Your Life " published in 2004.

Recovery and Set Back

After I left the hospital and returned home I expected a full recovery even though it would require time and patience. Though I lacked knowledge of details about the cause of the stroke or the residual affects, my expectations were for a full recovery. My lingering concern came from a truism spoken by the neurologist to the affect that my recovery would be whatever occurred.

For the first time I had learned how swiftly and unexpectedly one's body can malfunction. Each of us house a combination of cells, bones, organs, and blood providing nutrients and oxygen. All operate in miraculous balance. Of the trillion of cells each of us possess, millions die and are replenished every second, but brain cells including the inner brain cells in the thalamus appear not to replenish or to be replaced by healthy tissue when there are injured cells.

Our physical health protects us until age begins to erode the body's defense mechanisms, or foreign matter attacks the body and is not attacked by the body's normal defenses, or an injury or illness destroys or breaks down a vital body function. The danger from damage to the brain is the limited ability for the brain to heal the damage or to compensate with other parts of the brain adopting the functions previously controlled by the now injured cells.The right and left cerebellum can have such capability. I had had the benefit of good health for my entire life. So any moments of pessimism I felt, I put aside. I was confident that I had only suffered a period of temporary weakness and discomfort. I was wrong.

73

As I look back, I had not asked the specialists the tough questions. I would have to learn on my own without an introductory course from any of my physicians. My family had even less knowledge. Because there are no longer any house calls, the specialist or GP who continues to see the patient should require the closest member of the family to be present at the first appointment in situations of serious illness or lengthy recovery with a lengthy question and answer discussion..

Armed with knowledge, the family can help the patient cope with unexpected setbacks and help maintain a positive attitude. Each lead specialist today should allocate time for this purpose unless the family doctor has assumed the crucial role of central communicator. Such a discussion should be included in the preparation for the patient's departure from the hospital or during the first office visit. Such a meeting is an essential part of a doctor's medical role in the recovery process. This was a medical role that my father considered essential and now often falls through the cracks. Dad's house calls were partially designed to bring the family into the healing process. House calls provided dad with the ability to observe the home environment. He would make recommendations on diet, hygiene, exercise, and harmony. Often he became the advisor to help the family to understand and to cooperate in the healing process.As he was outside of the family and a respected friend he became a helpful advisor toward other family concerns that could restore harmony to the home..

Once I was out of the hospital and recuperating at home, my attitude reflected an atmosphere far more conducive to restoring the body's natural balance than I experienced in the hospital. I was able to sleep at night without the ever-present noises and disturbances interwoven into the nightly functioning of a hospital. I could start the day with a view of the sunrise emerging over the eastern horizon with a reddish glow on the waters of Long Island Sound. My breakfast was brought by my wife on a tray so that I could remain in bed till I was comfortable enough to overcome my reduced energy level. I would then dress. I had regained the ability to use my muscles. I had a normal sense of feel.

To reactivate my long-dormant knowledge of pathology during the first two weeks at home, I reread the books on anatomy my dad had given to me. I looked at the diagrams showing the arteries, which carry blood, pumped from the heart. The diagrams showed blood flowing throughout the body into more and more minute passageways to bring oxygen and nutrients, including the brain's billions of cells. The book described the nervous system as a system that transmits information and data to and from the brain. The brain was described as the controller, interpreter and activator, making use of a vast storage system known as memory, both subconscious and conscious, and long and short term memory. I was developing a new focus of concentration with the hope of understanding the inner workings of the brain through a process of self-education without physician input. My knowledge was limited by the publication date of these books.

My health began to improve. Although I still needed to concentrate to have my right arm and leg respond, the lack of muscle strength had slowly disappeared. My sense of feeling had returned to normal. My energy level gradually increased but remained at a reduced level. I could be active for several hours before becoming exhausted and needing to rest. My most noticeable mental limitation was that I would reverse numbers and letters without being aware that I was doing so. Each day there was a slight improvement.I would rise from bed at my usual hour about 6:30 in the morning. By leaning against the wall I would reach the bathroom. I used the banister to walk down the stairs. My breakfast reflected my normal appetite. As long as I was sitting I was comfortable. I could drive my car.

Three weeks after my discharge from the hospital, I called the neurologist and asked him what he thought of my returning to work for a few hours each day, including my ability to commute. His answer, as I look back, fitted the pattern of responses, "If you feel you can do it, go right ahead. " I have learned that as a patient, I could expect only a limited amount of time to be spent with me by each physician. Less emphasis is placed on the role of the patient in his own recovery and their understanding of the details of their medical condition.

The medicine reducing the odds of another stroke was the only pharmaceutical tool the specialists could offer me. There was no medicine to help my recovery. Because of the discoveries that have been made by the pharmaceutical industry, physicians either believe or know that medications out perform the body's natural ability to combat illness. The physician's understanding of the appropriate drug helped by the literature of the pharmaceutical company has supplanted my father's reliance on the recuperative powers of the individual.

Even the older current medical practitioners with a few exceptions have less time to focus on the patient, the patient's medical history, their inner feelings, their understanding and motivations. This was well said by Dr. William Duskash, the doctor to former President Lyndon Johnson. "I've become aware of the importance of knowing the ramification of the total patient, his personality, his dislikes, how he handles fatigue and disappointments, how he is able to be re-energized, and how all this affects his health."

Patients react to physicians with a sense of separation. A patient who tries to achieve equality in the relationship runs up against their egos, rooted in their medical training, financial wealth as the result of that education, and the status in society which comes with both. During emergency medical treatment the need to diagnose quickly through the use of technology and then to involve the right specialist can leave an incapacitated patient feeling totally left out.

Without fully appreciating it, I was in a period of psychological transformation. My illness brought an inner sense of solitude, a feeling that the residual affects were acting as a separator from my normal relationships. The concentration on the physical changes meant a new inward focus. Emotional I needed to sense that my family understood the new physical and emotional limitations but at the same time avoid expressions of sympathy. I needed unspoken support both physically and emotionally. My family and I were to experience a lengthy time period before either of us understood the real nature of the brain damages and the symptoms that they would produce.My wife sensed my withdrawal as I adjusted to the new limitations. The difficulties occurred in how to reach out to me.

With the end of my hospitalization, my recovery was up to my body's own recuperative powers. My physical recovery after my discharge was slow especially the restoration of my normal energy. For the first six month period after my hospitalization, I made routine visitations with the neurologist every two months at his New York office lasting 15 minutes each. I spent an hour three days a week with the local physical therapist strengthening the movement of my muscles that controlled my right arm and leg. I lacked a real understanding of the dangers of future set backs after suffering a stroke. My wife and children had even less understanding.

As time passed, I became aware that a recovery from a stroke was a very slow process compared to many treatable illnesses or injuries. To see any improvement, I had to look back weeks or months. Although I was slowly improving, I still had moments of a loss of energy. The tingle within my right hand and foot remained. There was discomfort in portions of my right arm and leg especially the joints. They felt stiff and wooden. My mind was clear with good memory and the same intellectual ability. My emotions were in a state of flux.

My recovery, which I had hoped would be completed in a few weeks, was extending into months. I tried to ignore the discomfort as I had convinced myself that I was slowly recovering and that I would again enjoy normal good health. During the short office visits with the neurologist, there was no focus on the sensations that I was beginning to feel within the inner joints of my right arm and leg. A burning sensation over the back that I felt at infrequent intervals, I was told to ignore. It would cause no harm. There was no psychological preparation for what later occurred. The damage to the thalamus did not appear to show up on the later MRI pictures. It could only have been discovered from a give and take focused on a detailing of my symptoms that intensified at the end of 1992.

The morning daily starts took much longer. I could dress while sitting down easier than standing. During July I would walk by the sea with my wife by my side as she talked about the local museum where she was a docent.

During late July I began to work at my office for a few hours. I derived satisfaction and self esteem from these few hours at work. I possessed a needed expertise as general counsel. I enjoyed the control that I could exercise over the conversational flow. Even though standing in one spot for any length of time was still difficult, I was determined to work part time. As soon as I was able to drive my car the twelve miles from my home to the office, I had returned to work.

By early August I was working four hours a day at the electric utility. I felt better when at work and concentrating. I had less time to dwell on my discomfort. Because I often felt tired, part of my usual work load was taken on by others. Nothing was said but my colleagues at work sensed the need and automatically responded.

My daily swims had stopped. I did not have the strength and found it difficult to step down the cement stairs to the beach. It would be one of several years without my lobster pots being set and hauled by me from my rowboat.

By late August my wife and I took our summer drive to the small house on Mt. Desert Island that her father had built in the late 1920s as a summer home without amenities. When I first was there before my marriage to Ruthie the cabin had only a well instead of running water, had a wood stove and fire place, and an outhouse.The most impressive design was the high V ceiling of the studio living room. The windows allowed a north light.Over the years a pump station and a full bathroom had been added. An electric stove and refrigerator altered the summer life style. The most important healing qualities at the cabin was the quiet and the ocean view. I was unable to walk distances or climb the mountains. I could not pick the wild blue berries growing on the mountain tops. Ruth brought them at the market. We went to Echo Lake near Beach Cliff. The water was calm and shallow. There was a rope that divided the water where the depth increased. I slowly walked into the lake. Buoyed by the water I swam a short distance with a slow over hand stroke. I had the wonderful feeling of reaching a new phase in my recovery. At night Ruth and I enjoyed boiled lobster watching the frigid Maine waters in front of the cabin. After ten days my wife drove the distance back to New London.Even with my physical limitations, I enjoyed each day convinced I was moving forward in my recovery.

The neurologist gave me limited information during this recovery period and his comments were repetitive. The other specialists had all ruled out as sources of my stroke any problems with the organs or body functions within their expertise. I no longer saw any specialists other than the neurologist and the hematologist, the latter because a blood clot had occurred.

Testing showed the blood flow through the carotid artery at normal velocity. The vertebral left artery during one doppler test indicated a slight slowing in the velocity flow, an indication of some plaque accumulation which I assumed could be due to my age. My symptoms, as opposed to the graphs and pictures from technology, continued to indicate residual damage. When I discussed with the neurologist the amount of time for full recovery, he gave me no hint that there could be any latent factors that might stop my recovery or reverse it. Not enough time was spent to get inside the patient. The delayed symptoms that I may have had damage within the thalamic portion of the brain began eight months after my stroke when the nerves rejuvenated. The patient needs knowledge and understanding so that if the pessimistic alternatives become the reality, he is prepared to fight to maximize recovery. This can only come about if the physician is sensitive to when there is the need to spend extra time with the patient. The physician can obtain necessary information not being produced by technology. Technology and a medical review of the images could not determine the cause of my stroke.,My delayed symptoms were the source of knowledge as to my brain damage.I did not have the symptoms till eight months after the stroke.

By late fall I had minimized the remaining physical difficulties. I believed that in the winter of 1993 with a full recovery my wife and I could travel once again to San Cristobal, Mexico, my wife to view the mountains and the beauty of nature as she sketched and painted, while I circulated with friends from a different culture.

These dreams ran into a new reality. All improvement stopped in late December 1992. Without warning, my physical discomfort began to get worse. Each new week brought with it a new setback. The tingle in my hand and foot increased. The sensation of hardness in the joints of my right arm and leg worsened. These changes shook my faith in my eventual recovery. Every day I felt worse. For the first time I lost my faith in a full recover.

The physical therapist was perplexed. She suggested I might be overdoing exercise. We decided to reduce my daily swimming in a nearby hotel pool and skip the exercises at the gym for two days each week. I stopped getting ultrasound.

On Saturday, April 3, 1993, I had gone to my accountant's office to give him data so that he could prepare my income tax return. I returned home at noon totally exhausted and immediately stretched out on my bed. As I did, suddenly the nerve system in my right arm and leg felt as if it was twisted, like the twisting of a rubber band. My arm and leg tingled. My anxiety level soared. Even with the deterioration since

December, this episode was frightening. I called the neurologist at his home and told him what had just happened. After listening patiently to my monologue, he suggested a switch from coumadim to tyclid and said he would call in the recommended dosage to the pharmacy. I did not know from his explanation whether tyclid was to help alleviate my physical discomfort or to help prevent a second stroke. It does the latter.

My optimism slowly disappeared as time passed. My attention was focused on the increasing discomfort. With no understandable explanation for the cause of the deterioration, my anxiety escalated into depression. Because my adult life had been rooted in mental discipline and a dedicated work ethic, I continued to work a half-day. By early April the discomfort and my focus on it ended my ability to commute and to work. When I stood in one spot for any length of time, it felt as if an iron rod extended from my right heel to the neck and through my right arm to the wrist. Only with concentration and thought control could I still walk and move about.

I told the neurologist the extent of the deterioration. He was concerned and recommended that I be hospitalized for tests and observation at Mt Sinai, the teaching hospital with which he was affiliated. By the time I entered the hospital my right arm would contract and almost withdraw into itself when I relaxed and did not maintain control. I had no knowledge or insight as to why this was happening. My lack of understanding magnified my sense of helplessness.

I convinced myself that my difficulty was due to nerve involvement that might be relieved by surgery. Without a medical explanation, I was unable to accept that the cause might be permanently damaged brain cells. I urged the neurologist to do an MRI of the cervical spine to validate a finding of damage. The neurologist agreed to order the test with little belief that it would reveal damage or sufficient deterioration within the spinal discs. It did not. I was discharged after two days in the hospital with no greater understanding of my condition and an escalating sense of fright. The only change in my medical care while at the hospital came when the specialist reinstated the prescription for coumadin and stopped the dosage of tyclid. Tyclid was causing a feeling of nausea. There was no discussion as to what my symptoms might be indicating.

The neurologist recognized I was becoming depressed, but his only reaction was to prescribe a small dose of an antidepressant, amitriptyline, to my daily intake of drugs. He did not suggest that I consult a psychologist or psychiatrist to aid the healing process. I had suffered physical damage.The neurologists were very conscious of the difference between physical damage to the brain and the chemical and psychological disturbances of mental illness.

I felt like a piece of medical garbage.

An Overlooked Depression

My depression and physical discomfort worsened. Weight on my right foot produced the sensation of an internal iron rod extending the length of my right side. I would tire easily I was most comfortable in bed. There were days when noise would create chaos in my brain. At other times a hissing sound would occur as a continual noise within my ears. My ability to maintain eye focus, to watch TV, or to read was limited to minutes. My subconscious mind blended with the conscious. I began to lose normal control and focus. I only felt comfortable with my eyes closed. Decision-making and activity were more and more limited to the fundamentals to maintain life : waking, toiletry, eating, drinking liquids, and more and more sleep. I found difficulty talking on the phone. Even that degree of concentration caused discomfort.

I lacked any insight into how and when my new level of discomfort and deterioration would reach a plateau. There appeared to be no turning point. I came to accept that my life's accomplishment had already occurred, making for a dismal future. I was not coping with my disability. Because of the difficulty of being with me in this state of agitation and remorse, the calls and visitors were reduced to two or three of my closest friends. My personality had become so withdrawn that my wife and friends had difficulty choosing stories and humor that would not increase my depression. There was no laughter.

I was in a cocoon, of sorts, but with no prospect of becoming a butterfly. As I became more depressed, I dwelled within the memories of my subconscious mind reflecting on secure childhood days. When

I would shut my eyes, as I often did, I saw a kaleidoscope of colors. My deceased mother appeared as a youthful vivacious woman in her 40s, an ethereal form exuding warmth and charm, a provider of early childhood happiness.

My depression was rooted in the uncertainty of the future and an acceptance of the closeness of death. The affect was to increase my physical disability. My depression reflected my difficulty in adjusting to a disability that was both uncomfortable and restrictive of physical and mental activity, or so I thought. My will collapsed. I lacked the knowledge to fight. A mind that had been trained on the importance of each detail knew none of the details causing my condition. There was no ability to organize them for understanding. My friends became alarmed. My wife and children were perplexed. They had never been exposed or had to deal with me as I now was. I had always been organized and strong minded. I had enjoyed challenges. If such character and mental traits still existed, they were dormant. The neurologist had spoken of occasional setbacks, but not a fall through three floors into a darkened basement. My condition went beyond my most pessimistic assumptions. I was confused. I had no explanation of what was happening. Why had I improved for six to eight months and then suffered such a reversal? I had forgotten the underlying force of the necessity to fight for survival. No one had explained that disability need not mean being non functional. Like pain it can be controlled but it requires motivation as the Greek philosophers understood by including Anarke, the force and Goddess of necessity, among their deities. The pull from necessity affects your attitude.

Disability appears the worst when the deterioration is unexplained and when confusion and a collapse of will takes control. I had lost the ability to accept my changed physical condition and to reorganize my memory to carry on the daily repetitive battle. I had yet to bring together an emotional strength rooted in the philosophy of my father that included the need to restore ones self esteem. I needed knowledge about my brain damage and the cause of the symptoms that I felt each and every day. Only then could I have a logic to fight my disability. My wife, Ruth, was perplexed by the deterioration in both my attitude and physical condition. She was confused as to how she could help in motivating any improvement.

Second Opinion and the Turn Around

I did pull myself together enough to seek a second medical opinion, as my wife and best friends had been repeatedly urging me to do. I made an appointment with a local neurologist to select a neurologist at another teaching hospital for a second opinion after a review of my diagnostic history. Once in the local neurologist's office, I summarized my condition in the few minutes that I knew was being allotted to me. Both my demeanor and recitation convinced the neurologist that I could benefit from an early appointment with Dr. Louis Caplan, the chief of the neurology department at the New England Medical Center in Boston. He called him while I was in the office and made an appointment two weeks later during June of 1993. I had been given a rapid appointment considering my medical problem is not and was not life threatening. Yet I had little hope. I went to Boston reconciled to another futile examination.

I arrived at the New England Medical Center with my wife and son, Philip, I sat down in a hospital wheelchair. I hung my cane on the back of the wheelchair and took the elevator to the 10th floor. I handed the receptionist all the technology: data, graphs and reports that I had brought with me. A young assistant neurologist saw me almost immediately and did a basic physical and post stroke examination. He also asked me a number of questions to learn the details of my symptoms. Soon after the chief neurologist, Dr. Louis Caplan, a specialist of about 60 years of age, entered the room. The young neurologist said his exam had showed no unexpected problems.

Dr. Caplan took great pride in his ability to relate to his patients and has written a book discussing strokes and the recovery process in lay terms that patients could understand. The book published by the American Heart Association is entitled *Family Guide to stroke-treatment, recovery, and prevention.* His approach was similar to that of my father. He was a humane, compassionate doctor, busy but never hurried. I realized this from his manner the moment that he entered the room. The medical visit had already taken an hour. Dr. Caplan took me to a corridor where he had hung graphs and MRI pictures of my brain. Dr. Caplan had been studying them while his assistant had examined me. He listened to the summation as his assistant verbalized his discussion with me including the spasm sensations about which I complained. He led me in front of one particular MRI picture, and asked, "Has any doctor explained in detail the damage that occurred to your brain?" I replied, "Except to tell me that I suffered a stroke that damaged brain cells. When hospitalized in April 1993 one neurologist mentioned the cells in the thalamus portion of the brain without any explanation.. I know little else."

Dr. Caplan chose his words carefully. "When you leave this office you are going to know what is wrong with you and what is not wrong with you. Because you do not understand your medical problem, you have become your own worst enemy on the road to maximum recovery."

As Dr. Caplan and I looked at the MRI pictures, there did not appear any unusual lines or dark areas. One of the May 1992 MRI pictures could be interpreted to show minor affected tissue in the Thalamus portion of the brain but the April 1993 MRI was clear. He spoke slowly. "My colleague's long discussion with you and your physical limitations and discomfort helped me to locate the small area of injury." He then pointed to an area smaller than the point of a pin. "This is within the thalamus area of the brain. This portion of your brain is where the cells receive sensory information communicated through the nerves. The thalamus is a staging area, like a switching network in telecommunication rather than a telephone. If you connect a new telephone and the switching system is faulty you will not achieve the expected communication. For you this means that there is nothing wrong with your right knee, foot, arm or hand joints or the regenerated nerve system. The damage was to minute brain cells, causing your current medical problem. The damage occurred because of a minute blood clot within the capillary artery feeding blood to these brain tissues. In the 1992 MRI there appears a very minor damage to certain cells within the thalamus. There may have been a narrowing of the artery feeding those cells but not enough to interfere with the flow of blood until a minute blood coagulation occurred. The cell damage is so minute that by the time of the second MRI in 1993 the pictures were negative. Your symptoms and history helped me to focus on the location. Once the nerve sensory system had rejuvenated over a six to eight month period, these cells were again connected. The sensory nerve cells have been giving out and receiving false signals. Your motor control is normal. The brain has restored the full strength of your right muscles. The brain had the ability to take full control of the right side. Over time you should adjust to the problem produced by the damaged cells within the thalamus. As the right side which suffered initial loss of muscle control and feelings and has recovered, only the right side joints have been affected by the faulty information from the thalamus switching system. "The spasm or twisted sensation creating discomfort and the feeling of an inner hardness within the joints of the right arm and leg are false information being given off by the damaged cells. This can occur when cells within the thalamus are damaged. You must fight to recover each and every day. In a sense, you must fight your own brain."

Dr. Caplan said he recommended switching my medication from coumadin to one coated aspirin a day. He gave me samples of an antidepressant. My local doctor would determine when it was at the right level. He said that when taking a coated aspirin daily my blood would not have to be tested, as required when taking coumadin. I would avoid the danger of bleeding if I cut myself, which is a side effect of coumadin. " For you, either medicine results in the same odds of protection against another stroke. " I was about to leave the office. Dr. Caplan reached out and grabbed the wheelchair. "This is hospital property. It stays here," he said. I rose from the wheelchair with the help of my cane. Dr. Caplan grabbed the cane. "I know someone who needs this cane, you do not. Now, walk to your car." I did. My wife and son walked along on each side of me as we returned to our car. I noticed each of their mouths were slightly opened with a sense of relief and hope.

The examination and discussion took nearly two hours. Clearly, Dr. Caplan understood my father's approach to medicine. Both men understood the role of an educated patient and knew that his or her knowledge and motivation was an essential part of the curing process. This is most true if the patient has a disability with which he must learn to cope. I was beginning to understand that I had to accept the fact that the diagnosis of brain cells damage (pathological damage) was correct and that it had resulted in permanent damage including pain discomfort.

This understanding of the underlying details that were causing my discomfort was crucial. I began to improve immediately. My survival instincts took hold. Over the next few weeks my depression subsided. I had the will to survive and to improve my health. Prior medical conclusions other specialists had articulated were correct; but they had failed to provide me with either understanding or motivation. Because this did not occur, the result was a breakdown of the curing process. Once a specialist finally helped me to understand the medical condition I faced, the will to recover reasserted control. It gave me the psychological tools I needed to end my depression along with an increased dose of an antidepressant as a catalyst.

I began immediately to act on Dr. Caplan's advice. The next Tuesday I shocked the physical therapist, who had been helping me at home with exercises. The exercises assumed that I was limited to being in a bed or a comfortable chair. On the previous Thursday she had demonstrated such exercises while I sat in the comfortable chair in the study on the second floor. She had left a pamphlet showing the exercises I could do while sitting.

The therapist rang the doorbell that Tuesday expecting my wife to open the door. That did not occur. When I heard the bell, I slowly stood up from my chair and walked down the stairs using the railing to steady myself. I then slowly walked to the door and opened it for the therapist. She looked surprised and a little confused. Half jokingly I told her I had flown to the Cathedral at Rheims and a miracle had occurred. We sat down and I outlined the events of the *real* miracle. My father's faith in the power of patient understanding, and his medical philosophy of mind over matter, had reasserted itself. I told her that Dr. Caplan had given me enough information, easily understood, about my medical condition that my confidence was restored. She and I spent the rest of the visit discussing exercises that I could do on my own while standing, sitting or lying down.

The Battle to recover and the Limitations

Now that I understood the true extent of the damage to my brain cells, I began to separate the discomfort and physical limitations that were caused by brain damage from the deterioration I was experiencing rooted in depression and anxiety. Although the line was blurred, I felt less depressed. Shutting my eyes no longer produced vivid colors and the protective faces of early family life and loved ones. I only eliminated my visibility. I accepted the probability that the one and only stroke I had experienced was not going to significantly hasten my death. The discomfort and hardness within my right arm and leg that were continually transmitted by the damaged brain cells was no longer frightening. If I increased my activity or stood for a time it was a conscious trade off of activity versus discomfort. I could decide when the activity was worth the discomfort. As time passed I slowly increased my tolerance for the discomfort. My will could again exercise control. I was able to stop all antidepressants.

Once out of the depths of depression, my partial recovery began, but it has been up and down and never complete. Although I understood the challenge, I did not know and received little guidance as to the length of time for improvement to take hold or to the extent the discomfort would remain. The specialists treat each individual suffering from brain damage as unique, limiting their guidance. They know each patient will have different resources and tolerance for discomfort. Specialists know there are millions of cells and even with the imagery and grafts from technology were unsure of the extent of the damage. They offered little guidance as to the future. Silence seemed for them a better tool than the ego difficulty of admitting they did not know. The standard practice was to refer me to physical therapy. There was little change in the advice or explanation in my regular neurological physical exams, six months apart. I continued to ask for new appointments until I came under the care of Dr. Lloyd Saberski, a pain specialist in New Haven.

I would have begun the battle for my own recovery earlier and suffered far less mental trauma if the earlier specialists had treated me as an equal partner and filled in the voids in my understanding.

I might have avoided the attitude that I was medical garbage.

In my father's day, fifty years ago more lives were lost, the curing process was more difficult, and the doctors lacked the magic of drugs. Doctors regarded patients as their congregation in much the same sense a rabbi, minister or priest might feel toward those to whom they minister. They felt a responsibility as a physician to each individual patient to unlock their inner resources to join in the recovery. It was this lasting impression from my childhood that had given me expectations that I should have logically known that the medical profession has difficulty meeting today.

By June of 1994 I had recovered enough to resume outside social activities. The equinox and solstice celebrations with the Merrill were held at our home on June 21st. We toasted the start of each season in recognition of a ceremonial faith in the sun's yearly journey. The party every six months was held at our home with one uncertainty. I would bake popovers and was never certain until I removed them unstuck from the pan of my success. I broke into a big smile that spread to everyone as they knew the buttery taste of my best popovers would soon be enjoyed. These small successes were I hope the stepping stones in my walk to a restored self esteem and a future of pleasant moments of contributions.

I had to adjust to both retirement and spasm disability. I was unwilling to remain idle at home. I wanted more activities than physical therapy. Physical therapy without other activities was a route to irritability and frustration.. I had to reach out to prevent the loss of ego. With a lifetime involved in a work ethic, the home environment would not by itself restore a positive emotional attitude. Three of our children were raising their own families at homes distant from ours. Anna had adjusted to living in Vermont. My wife when not painting was reaching out to use the arts as a tool to educate children both at the museum and at the elementary schools.

Despite an attitude against a retirement in Florida, my wife and I had found a unique condo development within a nature preserve on the west coast of Florida at Sarasota.. The natural environment was retained so that many of the condominiums were hidden from view. The atmosphere attracted retired teachers and artists. My wife hoped to enjoy the other artist residents. After a visit we decided to live there three winter months each winter. They had a teaching University. I began to teach a weekly course on the interconnected global world and the consequences of the loss of the super power status of the United States. I did research about China as an emerging nation of power.

There were new friends as well as some of my old clients who had retired in the Sarasota area. I began to go to small gatherings,,joined a weekly retirees luncheon group, attended lectures,and musical evenings. When necessary I rested in the afternoon. More often I would swim in the pool or the Gulf of Mexico when warm enough.. Before the stroke my retirement thoughts were about travel to other cultures and to some of the locations of natural beauty to reinvigorate my curiosity and intellectual absorption. I was not now able to endure the constant motion of such travel. Life is both a series of compromises and adjustments to new plateaus.

The balance of the year was a greater challenge.Friends proved to be helpful. I enjoyed my social life.Many of my friends were still active in their business or professional activities. My advice as an elder statesman would be appreciated but without any real involvement.I began to write.

There were moments if not hours of frustration from an awareness that my learned skills were under utilized.My thoughts would imagine a use of my training. There were many volunteer organizations needing help that could use my background. The will to go forward was there but the spasms became an unwanted anchor. The reality had set in that I remained too uncomfortable. Like a young person looking to begin, I needed the opening of the door for a position structured to fit into my disability. It finally occurred.

My friend Tony Sheridan called. He was first selectman of Waterford. The town was in discussions with Dominion Resources as to the valuation of two nuclear plants that had to be assessed for Real Estate and Personal Property taxes. The generation plants were the highest paying taxpayers. The Director of Finance and the Assessor did not know how to value these operating nuclear plants in a competitive utility environment.Tony Sheridan knew of my background.I had helped to write the prospectus for the Bond issue to buy a small per cent interest in the larger of the two operating nuclear plants then owned by Northeast Utility. A small interest was purchased by the Cooperative when I had been their General Council..

When he asked if I would become a consultant, I immediately said "yes".

The next day I was seated in a room at the Waterford town hall. The three men from Waterford were all present. On the table was the lengthy document containing the prior settlement with Northeast Utility.The document was out of date. The settlement document was written before the end of regulations that valued generating plants on a reasonable rate of return for prudent investments. The value today is based on the so called competitive market place. I explained the marginal pricing system. I talked about discounted cash flow. I told them that the original purchase by Dominion occurred at a regulatory forced sale of Northeast Utility's nuclear generation facilities. The sale was below the current fair market value..There were blank stares.I began to explain each of the terms used.It was the beginning of a five year consulting arrangement.The town and Dominion attempted unsuccessfully to negotiate a settlement. The town had to litigate the issues before a court to a final judgment.

The activities as a consultant I performed when I felt well. The concentration required during the meetings ended most of my discomfort. I enjoyed each of the men with whom I worked. Tony was a friend. The others became friends.My fees helped to supplement my retirement income.A star had twinkled briefly to cast light on a finite period of time.

For a long time I accepted the fact that my brain damage was not of the type that could be helped by drugs currently on the market. My brain can not be trained to remove the malfunction of these damaged cells that cause the spasm Nor can the thalamus substitute new cells at this stage of medical research. I accepted the fact that all time would do is to allow for minor adjustments as the discomfort continued.

There remained a latent hope for an effective pharmaceutical treatment without serious side effects. In the meantime, each day I relied on my inner strength and determination to reach the limits of daily activity and to expand the levels of acceptable discomfort. I have learned to live within my present physical plateau, but it has taken a long time. I have learned how to live with discomfort every day. I now rarely see specialists.

I had one more moment of fright in June of 1996 when I suddenly felt a weakness in my right side and arm much like the night of my stroke a little more than four years previous. Instead of struggling to a couch or bed, I laid down on my back and breathed deeply. I did this for one-half hour. Then, full of anxiety, I tried to stand. To my great relief, my right side, arm and leg had strength. I immediately called the local neurologist.

Again, an MRI found nothing. The neurologist debated then, and still does, whether I had a Transient Ischemic Attack (TIA), a momentary clogging of an artery but not enough stoppage of the blood flow to cause any damage. My only reaction was a temporary switch back to coumadin and regular blood testing. If a TIA had occurred, it was while I was on aspirin. I know that the preventative medication is a game of reducing the odds of another stroke.

The breathing was a self-protective response. I did this to increase the oxygen in my system and direct the oxygen into the brain. I had in the four years since my stroke reached out to eastern medicine. I was looking for what answers it might have that western medical practice did not offer. I did this without support from the specialists, nor with any belief in its curative capability. Rather, I regarded Eastern medicine as an alternative remedy under circumstances in which I had nothing to lose. By exercising control within my brain I had learned to push the intake of air to a specific internal location with deep breathing. I had learned how to induce total relaxation with a foot massage. This combination had provided some temporary relief.

Weekly, I went to the home of the practitioner. When I entered there was a large room overlooking a salt water marsh. The room had a mat on the floor and there was a melody of relaxing music to be heard. After walking barefooted in a circle each of us laid down on the mat and breathed deeply. The practitioner then massaged the bottom of our feet. I felt completely relaxed. I was told to breathe deeply concentrating my thoughts to move the air deep inside my brain. As my mind was removed from my daily concerns and discomforts, a complete feeling of relaxation void of outside thoughts occurred. During this time there was more comfort. When I again put on my shoes and walked outside, the hardness again took hold.

At the same time I continued my daily physical therapy as recommended by my physical therapist. I swam every day and did arm and leg exercises in either a pool, or the ocean. I began my ocean swimming each year in late May when the ocean temperature reached 62 degrees. I did exercises and deep breathing before going to bed and in the middle of the afternoon. Over time I achieved a slow improvement with fewer moments of energy loss, a disappearance of sounds such as hissing in my ears, and fewer sunburn sensations on my back.

Alternatives to Medical Care

There was much I could not do. I could not push myself to take long plane trips that required sitting for a long time. I could drive distances by stopping every few hours to exercise and loosen the arm and leg. I often reached a state of fatigue within a few hours.

I was not satisfied with my progress. For these reasons I explored Eastern medicine. Eastern medicine emphasizes diet, natural herbs and breathing, and the reduction of anxiety through relaxation and the subconscious. By spending time reading articles in medical journals, I had learned enough about my brain injury to understand that the blood clot had cut off the oxygen flow and nutrients to the damaged cells. Eastern medicine believes in the need for a continual and expansive flow of oxygen within the body. I do deep breathing exercises before going to bed as a daily routine. I lie on my back and inhale and exhale drawing in oxygen and removing carbon. I relax with soothing music and with foot massages. They provide comfort which lowers the continual spasm sensations.

I was taught to balance my emotions by adjusting to the surrounding environment. My emotions were expressed by anxiety, concentration, grief, fear, fright, joy and anger. These emotions should be interwove into understood responses..The key to maintaining the proper balance is listed as energy control, intake of oxygen, mind meditation, and sexual self expression.. In the terminology of ancient China, Ying defines blood and nourishment. Yang is energy and resistance.. Resistance radiates out to protect the body.

The role of the subconscious in eastern medicine is to reduce the patient's anxiety and become conscious of their thought patterns. A practitioner of eastern medicine creates for the client a state of relaxation and harmony. Slow motion, music and soothing language is used to reach into the subconscious. Movement is defined as a connected activity between mind and body that can be slowed to achieve a sense of harmony. The language and approach of eastern medicine attracted me even though I was a skeptic. Breathing I knew was crucial to a healthy brain and important for the nervous system. A reduction of my anxiety and induced relaxation lowered the level of my continual spasms even if only for a temporary time period. In totality, this tradition of medicine recognized the wholeness, balance, and harmony of the living being.

Eastern medicine, with its roots in the ancient medicine of China and India, included the use of herbs and natural supplements. As a result I added oxygen-producing rosemary to my diet, along with natural vitamins, garlic (thins the blood), honey (B complex vitamins) and olive oil. I was once again taking the dietary supplements that my dad had learned from certain of his patients.

Permanent Disability

As I approached my seventieth year the emotional section of my brain had a new sense of loneliness. I had to spend time each day in the physical battle to maintain my health plateau. There was the passing into death of my closest friend for twenty five years. He had never stopped smoking. He had lived with the philosophy of wanting to enjoy life, help others professionally, and depart whenever it should happen. I know that the smoking habit hastened his death. I felt an irreplaceable loss. My two clients who had created a national retail corporation and who were good friends were gone. One had died from a stroke. There would be no more flights to Florida on the company plane as I briefly enjoyed the new opulence that was the life style for the selected few. Age reduces friendships and companionship. Although my body was never free from discomfort, I was still a survivor.

Over a period of time I made a conscious effort to reduce my idle time and to avoid boredom. I developed new friendships for lunches. I used my training to organize material and a lifetime of interest in economics to do consulting work in areas where I had developed a work expertise. I wrote financial articles to distribute to my contacts still active in their business or professional pursuits.

After my stroke and the damage it caused to certain cells, I have looked at my brain in a much different way. I continue to exercise it with thoughts and mental activities. The emotional section of the brain provides feelings of love, anger, anxiety, and enjoyment. However, I have added to these thoughts and emotions a detached scientific approach based on the current knowledge of neurologists but rooted in my father's approach to medicine. I have learned that the brain can communicate between the right and left cerebellum hemispheres. They compensate for damage cells in one sphere by substituting active live cells in the opposite sphere. Over time it restores the functions to control muscle strength. This may take many months and continual effort but it can be a functional result with certain patients. I was fascinated by this knowledge of the brain's ability to adapt and to substitute the functions of certain injured cells.

My brain had the ability to restore strength and feeling to the right side in a very short period of time. Those cells fortunately had not been permanently damaged and needed but a short period of recuperation and daily therapy. There was no need to borrow from the opposite hemisphere.

Medical books and articles taught me that the brain consists of a number of sections each one performing a different function. As the brain cannot store energy, it needs constant replenishment of oxygen and nutrients through the flow of blood. The heart, the body's pumping station, sends 1/4 of our blood supply to the brain using four main arteries -- two carotid and two vertebral. The blood bringing oxygen and nutrients to the brain passes through these 4 main arteries that need to be clear of plaque. These arteries break down into multitudinous capillaries that bring blood to all the brain cells. A failure of the blood flow quickly damages or destroys brain cells.

The cerebellum sections of the brain are the input and output controller. They coordinate muscles and balance, receive information. They decide and instruct. The limbic system affects the emotional life that includes the formation of memory and the sex drive. The cerebellum two hemispheres can communicate with each other and may compensate overtime for one hemisphere's loss including the loss of speech.. Each hemisphere controls the muscle strength on the opposite side and one of the spheres controls speech. Right handed people control their speech on the left side of the brain and left handed the opposite. To restore speech is a slow and difficult undertaking. The frontal lobe is for decision-making. The hypothalamus performs the functions of smell, hunger, thirst, response to pleasure, sexual satisfaction. The hippo campus moves memory from short term exposure to long term storage The thalamus directs information (a switching station). Damage in this area can also cause a continual pain spasm and in my case a stiffening and hardening of the joints of the right arm fingers and leg and toes causing continual discomfort. The brain functions through neurotransmitters classified as information carriers..Certain brain chemicals can affect attitudes and mental balance. Since the time of these early readings of articles in the mid 1990s about the brain, scientific insights into the brain have achieved even more knowledge

Knowledge of my condition has allowed me to make the necessary adjustments in my daily activities and to maintain my self esteem. I regret but am not bitter about the lengthy delay before I understood my personal medical problem. I was not medical garbage.

Even though only a limited recovery has occurred, I have learned how to cope with my disability. I have a sense of relief by doing repeated physical movements of my right arm and leg.These movements produce psychological improvement rather than a physical change in the discomfort level. I try to ignore the feeling of discomfort being produced by my brain's injured cells and the loss of the ability of the nervous system to intercept pain as well as transmit pain. The physical movements aid my sense of confidence but have little affect in alleviating the discomfort.

I have learned that with total concentration, the brain becomes so focused that the spasms disappear. I can accomplish this by concentrated intellectual thinking or when I am emotional excited about a discussion.Both concentrate the brain and produce a positive sense of self-worth. When I teach a course I am free of spasm during the hour and half-period that I lecture and answer questions. When I swim I am comfortable but I have to concentrate to raise my right arm. Swimming blanks out your mind as a thinking and feeling organism. It is an enjoyable physical activity that provides exercise, avoids weight that hardens and stiffens my right joints, and allows me to establish my own time length and vigor.

Most people enjoy a period of partial relaxation. With partial relaxation, I end up with spasms as an accompanying sensation. I need total relaxation or none at all. Am I limited to a soothing massage, quiet music, a bowl of oat cereal (it may lower cholesterol), or sex, or to spend my time activating my brain into total concentration ? I have learned that daily activity both physical and mental increases my ability to function more effectively but with continual discomfort.

I awaken most days when the eastern sun's red tinted rays appear through the window of the bed room facing east. Both legs can move with the same control onto the floor. I feel the difference when dressing if I need to place all my weight on the right foot. The right joint becomes harder together with the stiff sensations that are continual.. As I dress there is a frown rather than a smile. I succumb to moments of frustration from the inescapable stroke damage. My acceptance of my health plateau reemerges with a widening of my mouth as I enjoy my daily oat cereal granola with a honey flavoring. My medicines are swallowed with orange juice. My mind begins to focus as I read the headlines and first paragraphs of the New York Times and the Financial Times. To organize my day I list the activities to be accomplished. My writing of articles uses the information organized from the Internet. I give my blessings often to Google and Yahoo.

The need for daily medications has made me aware of the modern medical world of pharmaceutical recovery. The patient and the physician must make decisions involving the curing affects and the side affects of the drugs being prescribed and taken. Drugs are not without side affects that can be adverse to a patient. A medical judgment has to be made that balances the recovery that the drug can achieve or its ability to prevent an illness against the patient's exposure to mild side affects or the small percentage of patients who can have serious side affects. There is a need to balance the compatibility of all drugs being prescribed often by different specialists The prescribing of a drug involves a trade off between these factors. Pharmaceutical companies promote the curative qualities of their drugs and down play the side affects. As the medicine I take will be a daily need for the rest of my life, it is important that they cause no side affects over a lengthy period of use. Because I was reading medical journals and articles dealing with medicines to prevent a strokes, I learned of a drug that had been approved for US marketing by the FDA. The claim was that it could improve the odds against another stroke better than aspirin or coumadin I began to take 75mg of Plavix each day. I was later switched to Aggrenox by the Veterans Administration. Both have the same ability to lower the risk of another stroke but Aggrenox is cheaper.Aggrenox combines a small amount of asprin with another anti clotting medication.

The drug, Neurontin, was prescribed for me in 1998 to be taken at a dosage of 1800 mg per day. It resulted in a lengthy but temporary period of marked improvement.

Neurontin reduces or changes the electronic impulses within the brain and inhibited for me some of the chemicals that transmit chronic pain. The level of my discomfort was lowered by this change to my brain's inner chemistry. I felt less pain.The spasm sensation and stiffness became more comfortable.. There was a lengthy clinical history of the drug Neurontin showing that it could be used for long periods of time without side effects. The original FDA approval was to reduce seizures. Anecdotal evidence showed that the drug might be able to be helpful with my condition.

Neurontin produced a degree of relief of about 40% to 50% against a discomfort level of 5-6 on a scale of 1 to 10. A normal healthy person would still have sensed continual discomfort, but for me it was a marked improvement. I was able to accomplish more normal activities each day. I could once again reach out.I had crossed back over the Rubicon as I tried to convince myself. My injuries would not be an inflexible line that limited my activities.

I called my son in Japan to say that I would make a second visit. I had last traveled to Japan the year before my stroke. I spent twenty hours on the airplane. I had no more than the usual fatigue.. I had arranged for a seat facing the bulk head where I could stretch my legs.

Japan was like old times.I walked my grandson, Robin, age 4 to pre school.He would run ahead and hide to confuse me. I located a tower near the school to know the proper direction so that we would arrive on time. I visited the school. Shoes were removed before entering the school. The children sat in seats facing each other surrounding a round table. The school was clean. There were no custodians. The children shared in keeping it clean.The first day they were told that the school was their responsibility. They spent their time learning to be socially responsible and to work out their differences without teacher involvement. I was impressed.

At night I learned the privilege of being the oldest. I was the first to use the hot bath, which is a large tub of clean water kept at a constant hot temperature. You cleaned yourself before using the hot tub. The purpose was to relax you for a sound sleep. I slept soundly each night..

I changed my diet. I ate more rice and less meat.Fish and vegetables were often served. Albert made sure I had an occasional dish of ice cream. My Japanese family joined me.

My son Albert had arranged for a trip to China for one of the weeks while I was staying in Tokoname..

In Shanghai we visited a Chinese medical school teaching traditional medicines. After our guide told us that Shanghai was a safe city in 1998, Albert and I took a cellular phone and toured by walking different parts of the city. We used the cellular for the guide to pick us up and move us about.

The most interesting exposure was breakfast with a Chinese communist party official in charge of tourism in Wuhan., inland from Shanghai on the Yangtze River. He referred to us as terrorist because of the recent bombing of their Embassy in Belgrade.His attitude reflected the official communist party line.The United States was too sophisticated technically to have made a mistake.His English was impressive.He had worked overseas for the Chinese oil industry including spending time in the Sudan and in Texas. He had learned English at a Chinese University and while in Texas.. He was proud that he had two daughters and not the usual one child, a son.

Shanghai at the time was an over built city. Pudong, the commercial center, had partially unoccupied skyscrapers. Tracts of land had yet to be developed. The elevated skyways, with four lanes on each side, were traveled on by very few cars. Development had exceeded the business, residential and industrial uses.The future produced the needed growth.

I had read a book authored by a Professor at Fudan University in Shanghai. The book dealt with the difficulties of migratory workers from the rural countryside. I had hoped to visit with him as he spoke English. I had no appointment. The guide asked enough questions to determine the truth of my request. His response was that he knew of no such University. The response was a lie. He could not bring a foreign stranger to the University without a pre arranged appointment.

The exposure to these different cultures activated my responses. I learned that I had an active and responsive brain. My interest in these discussions reduced my discomfort.

The drug, neurontin with its affect on the electric impulses within my brain had expanded my activities. I was able to reduce the amount of energy that I had to dedicate to living with my pain. The drug eased the feeling of right joints hardness Over time, however, neurontin lost its affect. By 2004 the discomfort would make me tired by mid afternoon. To restore the previous more comfortable health plateau, the dosage was raised to 2800 mg. At this dosage the drug caused drowsiness as a side affect. I lowered the dosage. I preferred discomfort to drowsiness.

In the summer of 2005 I switched to a new drug, Lyrica,400 mg., with similar chemical roots which had just been approved by the FDA. It causes no drowsiness. It has helped to eliminate much of the nerve discomfort. There is no improvement in reducing the hard, stiff and uncomfortable sensation affecting each of the joints of the right arm and leg. I still feel these sensations from the brain damage.

Living with pain at the spasm level has its own ability to teach. You learn pain has an environmental relationship. At times of stress, tension, worry, boredom, and frustrations, the level increases. Humidity can affect the discomfort.

With complete relaxation, and with feelings of accomplishment, excitement, laughter, intellectual exercise, physical activity and concentration, a greater sense of self esteem, the level of pain is reduced. With the brain in complete concentration there is no discomfort.

Because of the continual exercise routine, the greater concern about the foods I eat, and the elimination of alcohol except for a glass of wine, I am in better health today except for the discomfort than if I had not suffered the stroke. I resumed rowing my row boat during the summer. I pulled by hand the 2 or 3 lobster pots that provide a delicious addition to our summer menu when they were plentiful..

I have made more of an adjustment to my post stroke condition than I have to the environment that has evolved in the first decade of the 21st century. At home there were two grandchildren that lived with us for a short time while their mother studied for a masters degree. I can not comprehend the time that they are transfixed to a computer playing nonsense games or watching robots. My suggestions to read even with a reward meant the reading of a book about their games without either plot or creative language.

I was first exposed to economic values rooted in the New Deal which influenced my dad. I am disturbed by the believers in an economic theory that attempts to treat as a science their belief that economic growth occurs only from the accumulation and use of capital by a few, that can ignore the middle class, and that labels government as an inefficient and an unwanted participator. After the economic system nearly collapsed in 2008 and 2009, the involvement of governments became a necessity..The wealthy traders of Wall Street were determined that the government's role would be temporary.

I can not comprehend how the new integrated world will resolve the conflict between western private enterprise and government control or ownership of property and sources of energy in China. The rapid growth of China and India has occurred at a time that the developed world has just past through a deep recession. The control of energy and the cheap production of goods within China and India is slowly shifting the balance of power. I fear for the environment with polluted water and air. Global warming (CO_2 in the atmosphere) can affect weather, the melting of glaciers, the drying up of rivers, and the food supply.. I worry about those whose young lives will keep them on this planet earth long after I am gone. There is comfort in knowing that I am not alone in these fears. They will remain concerns till my death.

My days begin with and end with discomfort. I pretend that the future will provide some relief.There may yet be a drug that duplicates the improvement that I initially achieved from neurontin. Yet I have the inner strength to mostly ignore my condition. My father believed that each person over time has to adjust to his or her health plateau. I grew up having his thoughts repeated until they were an integral part of my sub conscious.

During periods of quiet and solitude my mind can not avoid thoughts of the alternative paths denied me, a retirement at a time of my own choosing,travel to areas of natural beauty, and an ability to replace the use of my learned skills with new constructive activities. I had hoped the vicissitudes of life would permit me as the next generation of my family to carry on with dad's dedication to helping people..

There is difficulty in reminding my family that my injured brain does not function with the normality that my controlled day indicates. Emotional outbursts cause an immediate hardening of the right joints. Noise and commotion create a similar reaction. The pain specialist refers to an extended period of household discord as chaotic anxiety. Such atmosphere opens my neurotransmitters. The result is to increase rather than lower my discomfort.

I have a daily exercise routine with occasional one day breaks. My meals are regular and hopefully a pleasant social occasion. I can read sitting comfortably or lying on my side. I can write with ease. Lengthy telephone calls and e-mails allow me to share my ideas with others. I have contact with. professionals and business leaders who were 20 years younger in age. They are still active as decision makers.

I still avoid a nap on most days. If there are evening socials or activities at the museum, my participation is limited to two hours combined with an earlier rest period.. I tell myself that the cause is the brain damage from my stroke. I still pretend that age is not a factor.

Friends passed on to others that I have a positive attitude after a stroke leaving brain damage and a partial recovery. Individuals and their families have called to seek help. Stroke damage leaves many sufferers and their families with great difficulty adjusting to the new limitations and the tedious path of recovery.

Those whom I have helped want to trust words of hope from one who has successfully suffered and fought back. I listen to the descriptions of the difficulty of living with the thinking brain largely undisturbed but with a daily reminder of the brain damage that causes difficulty of speech, limitation of muscle control, for others continual spasm or memory difficulties. There are frustrations as weeks of physical therapy have shown less than the desired improvements. They seek hope and an additional motivation to continue the daily struggle,.

Each visit in my house or usually their home reveals the multitude of difference from the brain tissues that were damaged. Most are right handed. If they suffer from weakness of their right side, the damage occurred to the left sphere of the brain and may cause the loss of the ability to speak beyond grunts or the blurting out of a short phrase.

How difficult it is for their mind to understand that the right sphere of the brain though not damaged must learn speech like a child, first sounds, then syllables and finally words, a slow and difficult process.

The functioning brain must stop trying to speak out as speech existed before the stroke. The mind must emotionally accept the return to the beginning basics in order to bring back speech through the process of brain cells substitution.

I recall my own difficulty in accepting damaged brain cells as the cause of the undamaged stiff or harder right joints. I hope to leave a house with family members more aware of the difficulty, more able to help and hopefully not impede. The patient often shows a more limited response as their eyes continue to stare and no smile replaces a closed lip of frustration.

Strokes bring about some of the most difficult plateaus in the cycle of life.

Reflections at Age 80

My father had taught me to devote a portion of my time to public endeavor or aiding others. As a doctor, his professional activities met his requirements.. At age eighty I must look to the past for the time that I spent in public service...

My youngest grandson, a joy to be with, was assigned homework to interview the oldest family member with the question, "What good had he or she done during their earlier life?". He was to write the replies in his notebook for school. My answers would have to be short as he would soon become tired of writing. I sat next to him on the couch. We cuddled together. He placed the board on his lap, took out a pencil, and was ready to write.

Fifty five years ago during the Korean war I had served in the army. I had been inducted by the draft. I had not volunteered.I could make few claims that would impress my grandson. The army was my first full time non educational activity. I had been sent overseas to join the army occupying Germany.This was a good start to the interview. His grandfather had spent time in the military.He had his old army uniform in the attic.

He told me that he was not interested in my work as a lawyer for people or companies.He wanted an outline of what else was important for me. I had no choice but to quickly outline.

With friends I had helped to start in the mid 1960s the first Bank run by and for the benefit of blacks in New England. I had served on the Board of Directors and for a few years was the Bank's Treasurer.

I had inspected run down properties mortgaged to the Bank.. I made landlords repair the roofs. A few had to hire exterminators to kill the cockroaches.

I had been trustee of a small private secondary school

I served on the Board of Hospice in Brandford, Connercticut when it started in the United States. Hospice was to keep up activities and spirits even when everything for the person was soon to close down.

I helped the many in Connecticut who pay their monthly electrical bills to reduce the dollars that they had to pay while still allowing the private companies a fair profit.

I had stopped electric companies from leasing streetlights to towns and cities without the ability to buy them with an anti trust complaint.

My grandson had one more question. He asked "I thought you knew a few people I or my teacher have heard about.?"

I did. You can mention a few but not to impress your teacher.

Abe Ribicoff who was Governor, appointed to the cabinet by John Kennedy and a US Senator, lived directly across the street during the summer time.We were close friends as were the whole family. Three other Governors Chet Bowles, John Dempsey and Ella Grasso talked to me when I could contribute and help. I could call a close friend who was Deputy chief of staff at the White House when Jimmy Carter was President. I had good friends who ran big businesses. I flew in one of the company aircraft as it headed to West Palm for a Directors meeting so that I could visit my dad in Florida..My grandson was running out of paper.I had completed the interview.. My right spasms had disappeared only to return.

My routine has a consistency since my 80ᵗʰ year. By combining memories, with daily exercise, by organizing my thoughts directed toward a finite outlook, and by having a daily routine I hope to hold off any further slippage.

I am a survivor at age 81, seventeen years after my stroke. My routine combines exercise and intellectual stimulus with grocery shopping and household errands.

My right joints remain hard and stiff. Most morning I walk the cement walkway protecting beach front houses from normal storms. Conscious commands from the brain are needed to move the right joints into a walking pace. I stop every few hundred feet, view the reflected colors of the morning sea, and move a short distance further along. If I become too tired from the hard right joints, there are wooden chairs in front of two of the waterfront houses where I can sit and watch the ocean.The water may be still and calm or have white caps when blown by a strong wind. Fisherman are casting for blue fish and black fish off the rocks. Any thoughts of joining them are negated as the rocks do not form a natural seat. I can not stand and fish. My walks are limited to a distance of about one half a mile, a change from the two mile walks when I was in good health.

On getting out of bed each morning I try to avoid a frown across my face. I open my mouth to smile. The days when my smile is relaxed, when I feel energized and more comfortable, there is a reciprocal smile back.After a "good morning" with the warmth of a caring voice, Ruth walks down the stairs to prepare breakfast.

Most morning I sit in the reclining chair in the upstairs front sitting room overlooking the water before shaving or dressing. To make me feel in control I exercise my right arm and leg into various movements that have no affect on the hardness of my right joints. For me the movements are a psychological positive.

Over time I discovered that if my day has a scheduled enjoyable activity the tightness eases a bit.Different moods affect my brain and the injured cells. Days of rain or high humidity have a negative affect.

Ruth is 15 minutes ahead of me in awakening.She has slept better during the night and went to bed earlier. My orange juice is on the kitchen table and the bowl filled with dry oat cereal.I have only to uncap my pills and pour milk over the cereal.My newspaper is next to my dish.

There is little comfort in the medical knowledge that there is nothing wrong with my joints.The hard sensation did not begin until the nerves rejuvenated and became attached to the damage brain cells, eight months after the stroke. The nerve message system no longer reduces the level of my discomfort. but creates a higher level of spasm. The miraculous balance and functioning of the human brain that we take so for granted, is no longer a description of my brain as it interprets my right joints.

I learned as a lawyer to dig out the details of a problem and then to organize to protect a client from any future downside risks. I started from scratch after the stroke.I read medical books and looked at pictures of the brain. I read about the neurological functions of each section. I picked out those medical books written in simple English. As I tried to read and digest, I understood why patients continue to visit their doctor even when there are no medical tools to help and the concluding remarks are repetitive.

I had learned that with concentration as when in animated conversation or when giving a lecture the spasms nearly disappear. The spasms give me the most discomfort when I am idle and not concentrating my mind or when I stand with weight on my right foot and without forward motion.

My days continue to make use of my knowledge of the computer and the software involved. The computer helped to restore a more normal life.I can sit at the computer table with the screen in front,and the telephone within reach on my desk.I do not need my glasses. I have a picture of my Dad as a young doctor on my desk. A painting of my daughter, Phoebe, holding a doll created by Ruth is hooked onto the wall.The Internet provides the search capabilities of Google or Yahoo. I have a library, information, and e-mail contacting, all at my finger tips.

The physician specialists both in neurology and in pain management have left me to my own devises. The repeated message is the need for physical therapy, whatever that means, and to develop my own methods of pain relief. There were no drugs currently available except opioids. They made me groggy. I decided not to use the drugs.

The aggressiveness normal to my profession, I subdued with a polite overlay. I brought these traits forward to suppress feelings of frustration.I begin each day convinced that the following day I will come up with plan B, one day without discomfort. That day has yet to happen.

I exercise without standing. In warm weather I use my row boat and swim. Maybe I can still pull my lobster pots with the rope hauled over the stern.I can no longer risk falling over board. In cold weather I have the rowing machine. I have found out that if I sit or if I am buoyed by water I am more comfortable. Group sports or games with an opponent have been eliminated. Exercise is in isolation.

As soon as the spring air warms under the bright sunlight I take off my sneakers and walk the beach barefooted just above the water line on the hardened sand. The sea stretches across seven mile of open water with Fishers Island separating the horizon. There are memories reaching into early childhood. I spent my summers at Neptune Park since the age of nine.It was here I first swam long distances. At the nearby tennis courts I improved my skills at tennis after my tennis instructions at Andover. I learned to sail.As I finished the beach stroll I wet my feet to discover the temperature.The water is cold. I walk back to my house.

As soon as the Sound reaches 62 degrees in late spring, I pull my row boat on rollers from under the house porch to the beach.I have a rope attached to the row boat to pull it over the sand onto the water.I climb in and row out beyond the rocks. I row to the locations where I will set my lobster pots. The beauty of the sea just after the sun appears over the horizon is a moral booster for me or anyone.As long as I am sitting I am as close to normal as my hardened joints allow.

My intellectual activities for each day ahead have a wide diversity. I spend long hours in research and in writing I am learning to balance my tendency to organize with controlled language to appreciating the importance of details that give an emotional understanding to my ideas..My son Albert spoke to me from Japan as we both have the Skype software. As an artist and writer he speaks with a tough critical analysis of my writing.I had to change my style from my life as a lawyer.I had to spend more time including inconsequential details The change would create reader interest. My style was to write organized factual details in order to reach thought out conclusions.He sent me by e-mails with a number of examples. I used the computer to write, to correct, and to change wording and style. I often think of my dad's philosophy and his advice to those patients that survived with permanent disability.

He had a belief that an individual had an obligation, to himself or herself, to family, to colleagues, to make a contribution to society and to maximize what could be accomplished on each new plateau. Seventy years ago pharmaceutical had limited significance. Most medicines did not exist. Dad knew that this required the physician to spend lengthy periods of time not only with the patient but with the family.He would attempt to restore confidence and to reduce the patient's repetitive conversations about the medical damage and to help overcome the confusion. He had experienced many sufferers. Dad would patiently permit this early adjustment stage to run its course. He would then begin constructive suggestions on how a patient and the family should use their time to accept the new health restrictions. Playing with grandchildren or cards were on top of each of his lists as first steps in adjusting to the changes.

In today's medicine, physicians can no longer devote the time or visit the patient at home. Recovery from my type of damage or a similar disability now depends on the internal will of the patient, a busy day, and the most effective use of one's time. I never figured out onto what plateau I had fallen.It varies with my attitude. Dad's message to me would have been the same as the final remarks of the neurologist in Boston,Dr. Louis Caplan. "It is your battle to fight each and every day.".

I remember my dad looking at me, as a youngster, when I was seated in his car after he visited a sick patient. Dad spoke with his usual authoritative voice. A week ago this patient talked about what his life was like months before.Today for the first time he told Dad that he had spent time with a grandchild. They had fun. He was looking forward to sitting up and reading. Dad beamed with pride. His long visitations had begun to produce results.

My spiritual strength was not connected to a formal religion. I realized that my daily battles required a spiritual inner self to help with the return of my self esteem and the restoration of positive thinking. As the forces to sustain life were interwoven with my own daily battle, they increased my positive attitude.

I had discovered previously unknown changes within my brain when I had succumbed and then recovered from depression.To avoid any repetition I again thought of the stages of slippage and recovery. My depression began because my health deteriorated without any new malaise and no physician had been able to explain why, so that I understood.As the discomfort increased I concluded death could only be weeks away.I had believed there was nothing the doctors or I could do to bring about a change.I had not completed my goals in life or I thought that I had not. My inner spiritual self was failing to provide an additional meaning to my knowledge of evolution and my own body's disappearance at death.My feeling of self worth was not prepared for such an event.My mind rather than dwell on these thought closed down. I had day dreams of my youthful past when life had seemed infinite.I stopped my relationship with the present and the present disappeared.I was not part of it. When I learned the cause of the right joints difficulty in language that I understood from Dr Caplan,I realized that death was not about to take hold. I would struggle but could succeed in having the advantage of my father's genes and a long life. With the aid of an anti depression drug I restored my psychological health in a month time.I stopped taking the medicine. I have had a lengthy time to dwell on any relationship between after life and the complicated and unique human brain.

When my friend, Charlie Poole, came to visit me during the days of my depression his facial expression showed the shock he felt. I had no sparkle in my eyes. My body was too relaxed. The separation between my being awake or asleep was hard to detect.He told me a few stories of what he had being doing. His boat was in the water.We could go out to Long Island and have dinner.My expression did not change. There was little movement. He patted my chest and took his leave.

Charlie was my most trusted friend and financial advisor.He had integrity and good judgment.He was the first broker to explain to me the spreads that occur between the quoted buying and selling price for shares of stocks. He would credit me with the actual price and not the spread. It meant I received more money and he less.He had opposed the President of New London Savings Bank, as a member of the Board of Directors, when they bought a Bank that was making more money with a higher interest rate return because it was loaning to more risky developers.In the Bank collapses of the early 1990s the New London Savings Bank failed.We shared office space till I joined a firm. We would end the extended work day with a drink across the street expressing humor, social plans together, and exchanges that could occur because of our mutual trust.

After my depression I needed to put together a way of carrying on. I would use my acquired skills, my mental training, and would make a contribution to others within the new physical limitations. Like so many turning points in life the Greek God of chance joined with Anarke, the Greek Goddess of necessity, to offer a partial solution. The telephone rang. It was my old friend Tony Sheridan, who was First Selectman of Waterford. They wanted to hire me as a consultant.

My house overlooks the Sound but is set back from severe storm exposures by the water front properties.Celebrities like my ocean front neighbor, Abe Ribicoff, had long ago departed. Till summer time it is a quiet neighborhood with many of the houses empty. The only occupants of my house with bathrooms and numerous bedrooms to meet the needs of the children during their early lives are Ruth and I. Ruth is busy most days at the Lyman Allyn museum teaching young students to appreciate art and to understands the importance that art has in education as their classes tour the museum.My days, after I was not called for my work as a consultant, are up to me. There is no office to drive to, or a piled up work load to tackle.

I came up with two idle time reducers.I used the Internet to research the new global interconnected world and its affect on political and economic relationships. It would be a never ending research. It was not without a purpose. I had agreed to lecture to a retirement community in a Florida University by name during the winters where Ruth and I were now spending several months.The lectures took lengthy time in preparation.Much of the material came from research using the Internet.I had files to keep the subjects of each lecture organized with a sequence. My task was to change the lack of comprehension from watching the TV news stations giving out sound bites and dramatic photographs on a nightly basis into an understanding of the political and economic changes affecting the listeners.I sat down during the lectures. There was a microphone to raise the sound level. I allowed interruptions if any questions wanted to be asked. For the least informed there was a break through to a level of understanding. My salary was to purchase a few books that were related to the subjects I taught.

This Book deals with my stroke and compares medical practice in two eras separated by fifty years. The book is a one person clinical study. The book was a new undertaking for me.Little did I know how difficult it would be. My legal form of writing lacked the style to spin out stories and happenings to interest a reader. The computer was becoming a new opportunity. I typed, corrected, erased, and read what I had written on the display panel. If I needed information or an explanation, the research was quickly accomplished using the Internet.I could forward drafts for editing.

We returned from Florida to the Connecticut shoreline in early April. After Memorial day when the sound's temperature reached 62 degrees, I began my swimming. It was a shorter distance than before the stroke. I swam half way with a crawl and half with a side stroke. I lingered in the water to do exercises. I would swim a distance of 250 yards.In the afternoon when I felt the need to nap,I would instead take a swim to wake myself.

I set up luncheons on a regular basis with three of my best friends. David Anderson had put together a government to government exchange in Moscow as the Soviet Union began to have contact with the west. I participated. Max Belding, my client from Hartford who now lived in Old Lyme, and Morgan McGinley, the Editor of the New London Day were my two other luncheon companions..

David always had a luncheon martini and talked about his weekly horse riding. We were both Yale and Andover graduates. He had a strong belief in the need for a greener society which we shared. Although a Republican rooted in his aristocratic family we had similar views and attitudes.We were both mavericks.

Max Belding continued to be interested in the financial world. He still played 9 holes of golf.Max 's friendship began when Society for Savings picked him to complete the development of the new small community of Rocky Hill because of his business background and integrity. Our firm in Hartford represented him He was a rare combination of good business judgment, a commitment to funding the arts, and loyalty to friends.

Morgan's weekly needs were to keep up on politics and to write the editorials.He walked his dog at 6:30 every morning. Morgan could tell ethnic stories with humor and the proper accent.He wrote in a newspaper's style with great skill.He was entertaining.

Evening parties or dinners were more difficulty as I would feel less comfortable during this latter part of the day. I scheduled very few.

The summer brought renewed friendships with the summer people. Alan Berger, foreign editor of the Boston Globe, lived around the corner. Each afternoon while he stayed in Neptune Park he would join me on my porch to discuss the events of the day and smoke a cigar.

Afterwards we would both take a swim. I near the shoreline and he beyond the rocks that jetted out fifty feet into the sound.

My routine filled enough time to keep me emotional satisfied. My work with Waterford had been challenging, brought me into contact with bright experts,and required the use of my intellectual skills. I acquired new knowledge.

My winters at Pelican Cove,Sarasota are helpful. I would have preferred to travel and to use my background in overseas activities. Florida winters were a necessary fall back.I was assured of medical care if needed. I would take my chances that we would enjoy warm sunny days. I was outdoors without regard for rain or sun. I swam in any one of the six pools within our condo development. We had a variety of social activities as the retirees tried to remain active. They were of diverse and interesting backgrounds. Ruth discovered a group of artists that had retired but were still painting. Every March they placed two recent paintings in an Exhibition within the central entertainment building.The Condo complex had over 700 units.It was located within a nature preserve with many trees and Spanish moss hanging.

Bill and Karen Watt, who were ten years younger, came from the east coast for a visit. Karen loved everything about Pelican Cove. She bought an end unit overlooking the mangrove islands, the bay, and Siesta Key. Ruth created a large oil painting of Pelican Cove including the bay as seen from their unit.The painting is located on the wall of their living room.

Bill who loves the game of tennis when played with the goal to win was not sure if the retirees were aggressive players. I could not contradict him.I assured him that a half mile down the highway there were tennis courts with a top pro. He attracted some of the best players in the area. Outsiders were welcomed.Over glasses of wine that evening we celebrated their condo ownership.

Ann Sayre also came and after two days bought a unit. Ann lived in Denver and after one more year at Pelican Cove she bought a condo near the desert in Borrego Springs, California. Ann's husband, Jim, was our first pediatrician. In his later life he had set up medical clinics for the poor in the urban area of Rochester, New York after he retired as a Professor at the medical school. When they were in Europe Jim had passed away after a stroke.Ruth and I now rent her condo.

My lifetime training created tools that I use to weed out and to organize information.

As we entered the 21st century there were changes. The chemical affects and the electrical impulses on my brain from neurontin lost their benefit. We raised the dosage but it made me sleepy. We switched to the medicine Lyrica of similar chemical roots. It was affective at lower dosages. 400 mg of Lyrica removed the nerves twisted sensation but had no affect on the hard joints. I continue to take the medicine. When I ran out of a supply for several days I found out it was helpful in reducing the discomfort.Without the medicines I would be in a worse condition.

We continue to travel to the Cape to Falmouth once each year during warm weather to spend two days with my cousin Al Wilson and his wife Helen.Al's father was my dad's uncle who was trained at Yale medical school, graduating in 1910. As Al reached his eighties the afternoon sail in his modern rigged sloop with navigational gear came to a halt. Even with all the rigging and navigating aids the boat became pride of ownership not ability to use.

I needed to preserve the moneys accumulated to create enough annual income to cover our conservative living expenses, the Florida vacation, have some funds for three of the four children who could use economic help,and to allocate $10,000 each year to maintain and repair the old house. I began to read financial data. I read reports by top economists. I received investment reports from financial houses with a philosophy that the recipient had to invest with them I ignored their advice but noted their analysis.I opened my own account with Fidelity. Commissions on trades were $7.50 a trade regardless of the number of shares.

Toward the end of 2007 I wrote an Article that agreed with the few who saw a forth coming bubble and the break down of the financial system. I put 75% of my money into short term US government notes. There was a new problem as yet unsolved. My income dropped off to near 0 as the interest rate on government paper dropped to 0.I was afraid to trade the stock market.The 25% I left in conservative stocks proved by March 2009 to have been a bad decision. The market collapsed with the breakdown of the financial system.The rally since March 2009 only partially restored the losses.

The Article I finished in November 2007 wrote of the distortions and leveraging that traders were causing to the normal values of stock, corporate assets, and housing.I criticized Hedge funds, Private Equity Partnerships and the traders that dominated the financial system. I concluded it could not last. I still have the document as proof of my efforts. I asked Morgan McGinley to form a partnership. He would write in the needed style using my intellectual prognosis. He did not have the time and it came to naught.The article was never published.

For the first time since retirement I was forced to spend my reserve moneys on a monthly basis. I gave thought to reinterpreting my spiritual being to decide that I was not bright enough to know what happened after death even without my body.I would have to project a shorter life to have money to leave for daughter Anna's support and more than the house to the others.

Ruth was well enough to schedule infrequent trips to New York to visit art galleries.Always she spent time at the Metropolitan Museum. She would stay overnight with her Bennington classmate, Marianne and her husband. I had in the past enjoyed their company but could not muster enough control of my spasm to undertake the New York trip and the running around.The quiet while I stayed at home eased the discomfort.

A significant change took place during the four month time period that Phoebe moved in with her two boys age 14 and 10 as she studied and earned a Masters Degree in teaching.The commotion, noise factor, and breaking down of harmony over a four month period opened my neurotransmitters. The normal brain adjusts to control pain.Mine does not.

At age 80 there is the need for a quiet home atmosphere.The 14 year old grandson had been affected by Phoebe's divorce.He had outburst when frustrated or challenged without his less matured mind understanding, "why". Phoebe brought a generation change in attitude. Harmony changed to noise, loud voices, and discord. I knew as the days continued that my spasms were becoming more difficult to manage. Each week I felt the slippage until after Labor Day when they moved nearby to the Berger house I walk with a cane.

I will continue to carry on with my adjustments to the aging cycles of life Even though the stroke has made a difference affecting the last

17 years, I still look back to a life filled with self worth and enjoyment.I look forward to staying in shape and retaining an active mind with Diet, Exercise, and Purpose.

After a Stroke - a Recovery

After a stroke whether you are a recovering patient, the family, or the physician, you need to find out and to discuss how the damaged brain tissues have affected the pathology and the emotions of the patient.

Most stroke sufferers have an opportunity for at least a partial recovery. They must first understand and adjust with knowledge of their medical condition.

Does a patient know more than the medical conclusions, not in medical terms but in language that he or she can understand ? The details bring about an understanding of the medical difficulties.Instead of accepting the physician's explanation, each patient must repeat silently each word and term so that they can repeat them in ordinary language to the physician. The patient and the Doctor must talk the same language with the same understanding.

The patient and their family need to ask a series of questions to learn the details about the brain injuries that brought about the medical conclusions. You and your love ones must discuss with your physician all symptoms felt whether significant or insignificant. You should not interject any judgments. The details of the medical procedures performed by the physicians should be discussed using ordinary vocabulary. The pharmaceuticals selected to aid in the recovery or to prevent new dangers need to be explained including the affect they may have on the body's chemistry. You should be aware of both side affects and compatibility with other medicines you are taking. You or your family must then ask the physician if there is anything new that has been revealed during the discussion that had previously been dismissed or not considered in the diagnosis. The medical diagnosis may remain consistent with the earlier conclusions but in a few cases it could be modified or changed. The result could be an earlier and more successful recovery. These discussions require a time period with the physician of one to two hours not a fifteen minute pass through.

Any changes that have occurred to your previous healthy condition must be written down and outlined. The stroke sufferer must rethink their daily activities. You need to focus your mind to maximize these activities. You begin by rearranging your thoughts and memory, make a conscious awareness of each physical change, and make an adjustments in mental attitude to reflect the current image of yourself. The purpose is to restore self esteem.

The physical therapists can develop medically tested exercises but the patient must develop their own routine. Most important are positive thoughts directed at coping. The adoption to a new routine will be a slow process over days, weeks or months. The new routine should include exercise each day. Part of this change will be experimental. The family's participation with understanding is essential.

The patient must direct their attention to an early start of each day. Your diet is important starting each day with a good breakfast and a balanced menu. An early morning walk or deep repetitive breathing or an exercise period of 30 minutes whichever is achievable. The combination of all three opens up an attitude to look forward to a new day to rebuild or to hold onto self esteem. If confined to a wheel chair or bed an exercise routine to meet the limitations of a patient's physical condition needs to be achieved. Even if there is a struggle and discomfort this effort must be attempted every day. There can be no closing down..

Each day must have a schedule to maximize mental and physical activity. The family or love ones are a crucial factor. The patient often can not carry on these daily activities alone. Transportation may have to be provided by others., At times help with body functions or the limits to memory. The family must learn the balance between an inclination for repetitive rehashing and normal conversational discourse. When to say stop and when to listen is an art not a science. Each family member must remember the purpose which is to build a sense of harmony not antagonism.

The patient needs to seek out stimulation if it is available. The ability to continue reading, to engage in conversation,and to write are positive fillers of time.The telephone can substitute for former social or job related relationships. Activities that can become part of a routine are important such as the daily reading of a newspaper, magazine, or the limited use of television.or listening to music.The computer with the Internet research and communication abilities at your finger tips are a break through to help a recovery.

Projects that consume time to organize and to complete are important. An attempt to record the oral history that is contained within each of our memories can produce a book for your family if not others. Consulting work pursuant to an agreement or only to satisfy the individual's sense of their present capability even if without a commercial market is worth the effort. A well balanced diet is important both to provide nourishment and good health.They are occasions for social conversations.. A conscious concern to avoid sweets, junk food, and carbonated beverages is vital to the new health plateau. A dish of oat cereal in the daily diet can reduce the cholesterol. Salads, green vegetables and fruit are important. Juices and liquids assure a proper level of fluids within the body. Meat, fish, rice and potatoes improved with garlic, olive oil and herbs in moderation are part of most American diets.Deserts are a form of emotional comfort but not needed to balance a diet. If medicines do not eliminate alcohol then a single shot a day can stimulate the heart in elderly people.

How did these suggestions work out in my own clinical history ? All of the adjustments that can help a recovery have been mentioned in separated sentences within different sections throughout the book but have greater impact as they are now pulled together. What are my current daily routines, including other activities, since my stroke ? Each morning I awaken when the sun rises through the eastern window of my bedroom. I permit a half hour of lingering. I get out of bed to use the toilet and brush my limited number of teeth due to childhood braces and my age. I check the e-mail for a letter from my son in Japan. I dress with the informal clothes that I now wear. I have to steady myself. I stand on my left foot as I dress.

I am now ready to walk down the stairs to the first floor and the kitchen for breakfast. My wife has the coffee brewed and a glass of juice on the table. We wish our day with a mutual greeting and smile especially if it is sunny. Clouds and rain are a depressant. My breakfast is orange juice,oat cereal, a bun or bagel and coffee followed by a banana. Each day the breakfast has minimum variety except for blueberry butter milk pancakes with natural flour on weekends. Maple syrup is a must. I have eliminated egg yokes except for the pancakes I eat once a week.

After breakfast and my sitting exercises, I walk for ½ to 3/4 of a mile along the cement walk by the sea. It is still a struggle because of the tight hardness of my right joints. I tell myself I will only pass a few houses.Then I increase the distance. I repeat the walk each day. Once back home I sit at a table while I outline my day ahead.. Usually included are food shopping, a stop at the ATM machine, a luncheon, or a trip to the swimming pool or the use of my rowing machine. In the summer I swim in the Sound, or row my row boat just beyond the shoreline. I still have two lobster pots that I haul by hand.

I read the headlines and first paragraph of The New York Times and the Financial Times. early each day. I make note of articles to read later in the day.. Each evening before bed time I do a series of exercises including deep breathing exercises. I enjoy a warm bath.

Until recently I would use the computer each day to work on this now completed Book. I have begun to write a second book pulling together political structures and economies, the affect of the ability to transfer wealth at the click of the computer mouse, and the concentration of wealth. Does the failure of political leaderships threaten our future stability or the well being of our grandchildren in later life? Will the book ever be finished ? I do not yet know and care less. It is to keep my mind busy..I use the material in my Florida lectures.

Information and data and are now at one's finger tips. Using the computer and the accompanying software and search capability provides a new dimension to both intellectual exercise, communication, and entertainment. I use Skype to talk to and to see my family in Japan..

As is true of many retirees who depend on their accumulated savings to maintain their life style, I keep abreast of the stock and bond market activities not only within the financial centers of the United States but world wide. I regret that the financial world has entered a period of trading not investing.I am too old to learn the impact of derivatives or swaps on the financial system. How have I avoided idle time and the tendency to dwell on my physical limitations or discomfort ? In the recent past since my stroke I spent several years as a part time consultant to a town involved in a tax appeal over the valuation of a nuclear plant. I had acquired knowledge on the valuation of a nuclear facility in a competitive environment during my law practice as a utility lawyer. With a correspondent for German newspapers and magazines, I participated in a weekly TV broadcast for one hour each week on a local cable network station. The program terminated when my colleague became too busy with his other activities. During the three winter months each year that I live in Florida. I give a weekly lecture series on the new global world, the undigested problems, the incompetence of political leaderships, and the natural dangers that we will be handing over to the next generation. When I lecture I have no discomfort.

Despite the daily effort required and the reorganizing of my mind and memory dedicated to coping with my disability., there is continual difficulty. I feel the physical and mental limitations of living with discomfort. The key to survival on the new health plateau is the will to fight each and every day. There can be no day without the battle. Each day my right joints refuse to feel any lessening of the hard stiff sensation. I know my joints are in the same good shape on the right side as on my left except the damage brain cells do not agree and never will.

Each of the 70% who survive a stroke without death or full recovery must take on the imperfect recovery battle. The need to avoid or recover from a depression can be part of this recovery battle. My permanent injuries are the right joints discomfort. For some it may be a loss of muscle control on one side, memory less able to recall from some short term memory and for others from longer term. There can be the loss of speech which I was spared by being left handed. Each faces an adjustment due to the area where the brain cells were injured..

30 to 60 % will suffer some degree of depression.If our intelligence and mind's logic have remained in tact then we are equipped to take on the daily battle, to maximize the recovery, and to learn to adjust to

and to live with the health plateau left behind. My clinical case history should help the 70% not to give up, to retrain their minds, and to accept their new plateau as another stage in the life cycle outlined so poetically by William Shakespeare in " As You like It "..

Two Medical Eras

My medical history creates insight for doctors, patients and the patient's family. My stroke has enabled me to compare 2 eras of medicine, current medical practices and the medical practice of my father over 50 years ago. I admit to a certain personal bias as I compared my father's approach to medicine with that of current specialists. This is not without an appreciation of the vast improvement in diagnosis and in treatment achieved by modern medicine, and an understanding of the limitations in my father's era.

The flood of new information about the body, its structure and how it functions is so overwhelming that a specialist today is under constant time pressure to keep up with the new information and new pharmaceuticals affecting their specialty. It requires use of the Internet for new medical data. To garner insight into the vast knowledge involved in other specialties would require even more study, using unavailable time. For most physicians, the answer is to request the involvement of other specialists as needed.

Time management is demanded by the Insurance Companies. The refusal of the insurance industry to reimburse doctors for lengthy periods of time spent talking with patients, however necessary that might be, and the pressure for the practice of medicine to produce the expected profit, all conspire to reduce time spent with patients. The economics of medical practice today prevent all but the most unusual and motivated physician from spending the time to relate to the patient as a human being and to focus on the whole patient..

Many patients avoid medical visitations if they believe they only have a minor medical problem as it may take weeks or more to obtain an appointment if their problem is not an emergency unless the appointment is the annual physical examination. The time constraints in treating each patient cause most physicians to make quick decisions and depend upon technology to interpret a patient's condition. A patient must learn to rehearse the information to discuss with the doctor before the examination. Otherwise problems that are not serious or life-threatening may fall through the cracks, or a minor medical problem initially overlooked.

Dad believed in being face to face with his patients, a personal interaction with a social equality. He would dispense his medical services knowing his patients lacked insurance coverage. For many in the modern medical delivery system, Dad's approach has passed into medical history. Despite understanding the legitimate causes that brought this about, I feel sad both for physicians and for patients.

In Venice, Florida a medical facility has opened similar to the dispensaries in my father's era. The Catholic charities in the Venice-Sarasota area of Florida opened a dispensary. Under the oversight of active Florida physicians, retired physicians from other states provide free medical care at the dispensary. Instead of young physicians receiving clinical training as was true 50 years ago, the dispensary allows elderly, skilled specialist to continue using their knowledge and experience to perform free medical care, a reassertion of the Hippocratic Oath.

There are new teaching methods in certain medical school that involve the whole patient, not just the disease or injury. The University of Pennsylvania and Harvard Medical School and other medical schools have adopted the Case Study method as a supplement to lecture courses to make the medical student in training more aware of the patient. These case studies deal with the whole patient, his or her likely attitude while ill, and how the affected areas may react or not react to medical treatment.

The designs of a few future hospitals try to incorporate the patients' need for quiet and self esteem while in the hospital. Private rooms are included in the design as important in the curing process. The inclusion of more private rooms, as part of new hospital construction, has not caused a significant increase in construction costs. Completed hospitals in Chicago and Little Rock are based on private rooms, centrally monitored. Insurance carriers are paying a flat rate regardless of the type of room. Such private rooms if properly managed and with monitoring through a visual screen have a slightly lower operating cost. There is the technology to monitor these patients from a central control panel with complete visibility of the patient and his bodily functions. This approach permitting private visitations and quiet will shorten hospital stays. Recovery is directly related to one's self-confidence in reaching the maximum health plateau. Insurance carriers may also benefit. Any cost increases in construction can be written off over many years. Construction costs are normally only 7% of a hospital's annual budget. Private rooms allow for more family participation, reduced exposure to infectious bacteria, lowers the noise factor, and permits a degree of individuality. There is a greater opportunity for patients to reassert their self esteem. The cost to convert existing hospital beds to such privacy is prohibitive.

The Dartmouth Hospital near Hanover, New Hampshire is another recent example of designing a hospital to restore the patient's health by recognizing the importance of the environment. The hospital was architecturally designed to provide the feeling of a spa inside and a view of nature from most rooms.

An article in the Journal of the American Medical Society discussed the impact of psychology on physiology.

Physicians need to help a patient have less anxiety, less fear, and more optimism and confidence. This begins with the physician telling the patient details of the illness or injury, expressed in a vocabulary that the patient understands. The patient's understanding and acceptance of their health problems helps in the restoration of health. Medical specialists need to break down the Chinese wall between mind and body, that divides psychiatry from the physical. The brain has an important role in the healing process. If the health problem will require a lengthy recuperative time or change the patient's health plateau permanently, a patient's attitude and acceptance of his or her physical condition needs to be combined with physical, surgical, radiological, and pharmaceutical healing. Physicians practicing in specialties other than psychiatry can not ignore the emotions of a patient. Brain chemistry and the brain's structure are adversely altered by stress, by lack of appetite, by poor eating habits, emotions, anger, lack of self esteem and defeatism and have a positive response to a good diet, laughter, joy, optimism, self esteem, and confidence. A brain able too retains its intellectual capacity can overcome discomfort with concentration.

I had to accept an uncomfortable health plateau. Over a year after the stroke I achieved a cause and affect understanding so that I could accept and adjust to my new health plateau. I am a clinical case study that the whole patient plays an integral part in the recovery process.

The knowledge and insight from two medical eras need to be interwoven to provide the best medical care of a patient. The result would lower costs by shortening the length of the time period that a patient needs a physician. Knowledge obtained from the patient could eliminate the use of certain technology and shorten the days in a hospital.

There is a need for a relationship of intimacy and trust between patient and physician. They need to spend time together exchanging information. The specialist needs to communicate with the patient in an insightful, compassionate, and understanding way. The patient, the specialist, and the internist become a team. They spend more time with the patient. The Insurance Carriers pay for the additional time spent as they discover that it reduces overall costs. The patient or his family learn that symptoms need to be disclosed not ignored.

Modern medicine needs to treat the whole patient not just the disease or malfunction. Physicians today can learn of this need by becoming more aware of how medicine was practiced 50 years ago.

Bibliography

A.
1. Interview with Doctor David Sussler by the Connecticut Medical Association Historical Archives - July 21, 1992
2. Interview with physicians - partial contemporaries : Dr. Fred Barrett ; Dr. Henry Archambault
3. Interviews with patients - Alfred P. Savage ; Iva Savage ; Otto Grant ;Edith Grant; Angus Park ;William F. O'Neil

B. Book References
1. Claiming Power in Doctor-Patient Talks by Dr. Nancy Ainsworth-Vaugh, Oxford University Press, 1988
2. Time to Heal, by Dr. Kenneth M. Judmever,Oxford University Press, 1999
3. One Hundred Days, by David Bira, Pantheon
4. Family Guide to Stroke Treatment, Recovery,Prevention,American Heart Association by Dr. Louis Caplan
5. Harvard Med. By John Langone, Adams Media
6. The Invention of the Modern Hospital, Boston 1870-1930 by Morris J. Vogel, The University of Chicago Press, 1980
7. Concise Medical Dictionary, by Nancy Roper, Barnes and Noble 1995
8. Disease of the Organs by John H. Packard, Henry C.Leas Sons, 1881

9. Self Examination for Medical Students by George M. Gould, MD, P. Blakistan, 1891
10. Dispensary by George B. Wood, Grigg & Elliot, 1845
11. Physicians Book Reference 1996, 1997, 1998
12. Medical Schools Vanderbilt University School of Medicine-Curriculum 1998-1999
13. The complete Book of Chinese Healing and Health, Daniel Reid

C. Newspapers and Magazine Sources
1. The New York Times April 18, 1999 - Hospital Competition-Private Room by Milt Freudenheim
2. The New York Times March 23, 1999 - Savory Diet that's Good for The Heart by Jane E. Brady
3. Harvard Magazine May-June 1980 Stroke by Mark J. Rosenberg
4. The New York Times Guppies can Save your Marriage by Kris P. Maher
5. The New York Times april 18, 1999 Your Mind may Ease What's Ailing You by Erica Goode
6. The New York Times Hospital in Crisis by Bob Herbert
7. The New York Time May 6, 1999 - Teaching Hospitals Battle Medicare
8. The New York Tim April 6, 1997 - Doctors
9. The New York Times May 27, 1997 - Neurons to Study the Mind
10. The New York Times February 10, 1998 Where Marketing & Medicine Meet by Gina Kolata
11. The New York Times Easing Pain the Hard Way by Daniel Felber
12. The New York Times A Doctor Discovers How to Talk to a Doctor by Zoev E. Neuwirth, MD
13. The New York Times December 2, 1997 - Quick Action Helps to Mitigate the Effect of Brain Attack
14. The New York Times November 22, 1997 When Foundations Chime in the Issue of Dying Comes to Life by Judith Miller

15. The New York Times May 4, 1999 As Heart Failure Wanes-Heart Attack Rising in the United States by Denise Grady

16. The New London Day December 3, 1993 Reinventing the Way Doctors Work by Robert Sussler

17. Somatics, Autumn/Winter 1988-1989 - The Somatic Consequence of Emotional Trauma by Richard Strauch Ph.D.

18. The New York Times 1993 Too Few General Doctors by Elizabeth Rosenthail

19. The Wall Street Journal October 18,1999 Making the Cut

20. The New York Times March 27, 2000 For Want of Soap and Water by Elizabeth Normal

21. The New York Times November 27, 1999 How Medicine became Just another Product by Daniel Patrick Moynihan

22. The New York Times 1999 Doctors are Reminded "Wash Up" by Emily Jaffe

23. The Wall Street Journal 2000 Researchers Note Risk in Genetech Stroke Drug (TPA) by Thomas M. Burton

24. The New York Times 1998 Psychotherapy Found to Produce Changes in Brain Function (Thalamus) by Daniel Coleman

25. Forum May 19, 1997 Once a Physician, Now a Provider by Richard G. Williams

26. The New York Times July 13, 1999 Doctors Rustling Bedside Manner

27. The New York Times, May 18, 1999 Nurses, Patients and Managed Care by Claire M. Fagin

28. The New York Times Study in New England medical Journal 1997 Technology is Ending Doctor's House Call Journal Editorial to Have Medical Schools train Doctors to make House Calls

1. Copyright 2006 Robert Sussler under title My stroke Reveals Two Era of Medicine

About the Author

Robert Sussler suffered a stroke on May 15, 1992 at age 64. At the time he was General Counsel to the Connecticut Municipal Electric Cooperative that provided electric power for five Connecticut municipalities. He served in the military from 1952 to 1954. He is a graduate of Phillips Academy Andover, Yale University and Northwestern Law School. From 1954 till his stroke he practiced law in Connecticut specializing in Financial matters, Corporate Law, Commercial Real Estate,, and Utility Law. After understanding the damage from his stroke he became a consultant evaluating Nuclear Generating Facilities from 1999 to 2004 and a lecturer.

He is now retired. His wife for 54 years in an artist. They have four children and seven grandchildren.